Gender, Health, and Society in Contemporary Latin America and the Caribbean

Gender, Health, and Society in Contemporary Latin America and the Caribbean

Edited by
Ronnie Anthony Shepard
and Shir Lerman Ginzburg

LEXINGTON BOOKS
Lanham • Boulder • New York • London

Published by Lexington Books
An imprint of The Rowman & Littlefield Publishing Group, Inc.
4501 Forbes Boulevard, Suite 200, Lanham, Maryland 20706
www.rowman.com

6 Tinworth Street, London SE11 5AL, United Kingdom

British Library Cataloguing in Publication Information Available

Library of Congress Cataloging-in-Publication Data
Names: Shepard, Ronnie, editor. | Ginzburg, Shir Lerman, editor.
Title: Gender, health, and society in contemporary Latin America and the Caribbean / edited by Ronnie Shepard and Shir Lerman Ginzburg.
Description: Lanham : Lexington Books, [2019] | Includes bibliographical references and index.
Identifiers: LCCN 2019021105| ISBN 9781498572842 (cloth) | ISBN 9781498572859 (ebook)
Subjects: | MESH: Gender Identity | Sexuality—ethnology | Social Determinants of Health—ethnology | Social Discrimination—ethnology | Sexual and Gender Minorities—psychology | Latin America | Caribbean Region
Classification: LCC RC556 | NLM WM 617 | DDC 362.196/8583—dc23
LC record available at https://lccn.loc.gov/2019021105

Contents

Acknowledgments

The creation of this volume was a labor of love (and patience!), and it would not have been possible without a team of very supportive people. We would like to thank the faculty and staff in the University of Connecticut Department of Anthropology for guiding us through our careers from our start in graduate school, and for fatefully giving us an office to share. We would also like to thank the organizers of the 5th Queering Paradigms International Conference held at FLACSO Sede-Ecuador, which we attended in Quito in 2014, for accepting our presentation, as it formed the early framework for our co-authored chapter in this volume. Reflection on that presentation through text messaging—as we were each in gyms in different states—led to the development of the book in your hands today. We're eternally grateful to Chandler Burr, whom we have never met, for both his courage and inspiration.

Ronnie Anthony Shepard would like to offer heartfelt thanks to El Instituto: The Center for Latin American and Caribbean Studies at the University of Connecticut for his early graduate training in Latin American Studies, funding through Tinker Foundation research grants, and for all the *HACHA* social gatherings giving Latin Americanists a space to share their research and experiences. He would also like to thank his advisory committee, Drs. Françoise Dussart, Jocelyn Linnekin, and Samuel Martinez, as well as Dr. Blanca Silvestrini for guidance throughout his graduate career and feedback on the research that became chapter 3 of this book. He is indebted to the Torres family of Quito, Ecuador for taking in a strange guy in the middle of the night and always making him feel at home. He would also like to acknowledge Shan-Estelle Brown and Rebecca Rodriguez for their advice and friendship throughout graduate school, and their ability to be a sounding board for research and a place to vent on a moment's notice. He would like to thank his family, especially his mother Janine and grandfather Lawrence, for all their support, and anyone who has given him a ride to the airport for last-minute trips into the field. Finally, he would like to thank his grandmother Gloria, for asking every single day as he came home, well into adulthood, "How was school today?"

Shir Lerman Ginzburg would like to thank Igor Ginzburg for his love and patience. She would also like to thank Dr. Pam Erickson and Dr. Merrill Singer for guiding her during her formative early-career years to think more critically as a medical anthropologist, and to Dr. Stephenie Lemon, Dr. Milagros Rosal, and Dr. Laurie Bauman for providing her with valuable feedback through the editing stages.

Introduction

Gender, Health, and Society

Ronnie Anthony Shepard
and Shir Lerman Ginzburg

This volume takes an intersectional approach to the contemporary peoples of Latin America, the Caribbean, and the Latinx population of the greater diaspora. Particularly, the authors have used case studies, ethnographic research and data-driven theoretical approaches to craft locally-defined cultural critiques of gender and health in contemporary subaltern societies. Some of the central tenets in the crafting of this volume, and critical to its creative significance and contribution, are the conceptual unification of gendered health, the embodiment of identity, societal structures and social inequality, and the ways in which gender, health, and society intersect on a daily basis. The authors position subaltern identities, health, and well-being within personal, local, and cultural milieus that emphasize the complex ways in which gender is perceived and enacted. In particular, the multiple and overlapping spheres of gender and health identities in Latin America and the Caribbean are of interest due to both the marked disparities in health, economic, occupational, educational, and political outcomes between the genders, and also due to the Latinx diaspora and general movement of people that makes these overlapping spheres simultaneously visible and hidden, while also highlighting the incongruent ways in which different genders are constructed and enforced in the public and private spheres.

As scholars, we consider and question how various Latin American societies embrace or contest non-traditional performances of gender, masculinities, and femininities. When sexual identity is included, social scientists argue, it becomes a global dimension of power in which certain groups are privileged over others (Cantú 2003). Here we find that what it means to be a man or woman is bound in both time and space, ever evolving, and influenced by outside forces. However, those same outside forces often oversimplify the relationships between genders and sexual identities in Latin America down to a single word: *machismo*. Machismo too often becomes a catch-all to describe the behavioral patterns of Latin American males, no matter how misguided or generalized. While it is true machismo is related to masculinities and masculine performativity, it is only one small part of socially constructed masculinities and often does not apply in localized contexts. Therefore, the experiences of the male informants included in the following chapters should not be considered as signifiers of a rising machismo sentiment in the region, but rather as descriptors of culturally localized masculine performance.

This volume also considers localized forms of gendered health in Latin America and the Caribbean. Here, we find that the intersection of gender and health can be found in multiple points in society as signifiers of physical, mental, and social well-being. Some examples, which are explored further in this book, include: reproductive decision making and abortion access in Puerto Rico in the face of the Zika epidemic; the relationship between gendered parentage, same-sex partnerships, and the adoption of Andean children with special needs; and the impact of gender and ethnicity on treatment-seeking behaviors for sickle-cell anemia in Guadeloupe, among myriad others. In addition, social inequality is often a signifier of social well-being, and as such the authors consider the ways in which contemporary Latin Americans have adapted impoverished lifestyles to fit into an ever-increasingly globalized world. Situating health within and around these regularly gendered identities is often driven by quotidian social factors such as religious and moralistic beliefs and political and legal roles, as well as specific forms of discrimination and the intersections of multiple marginalities. These include stigma, poverty, racism, (un)employment, (dis)ability, differential wages, and intimate partner violence.

Gender and health have been proven to interact in a variety of direct and indirect examples. For example, obesity outcomes differ between girls and boys of Mexican descent, although immigration and generational status (e.g., first generation vs. second generation in the United States) mediated these outcomes (Frisco et al. 2016). Furthermore, gay, lesbian, and bisexual Latinos in the United States are at higher risk of negative mental health outcomes (such as depression), illicit drug use, and a lifetime diagnosis of sexually transmitted infections than are heterosexual Latinos (Martinez et al. 2017). Male health risks are attributed more to lifestyle choices (e.g., smoking, alcohol, injuries), while female health risks are attributed more to hormonal changes (Baker and Shand 2017). Indirectly, women are frequently excluded from schooling and participation in public life on a global scale, which in turn impacts their health literacy and informed decision making (Vlassof 2007).

Women's experiences in Latin America tend to differ depending on ethnicity, age, immigration status, urban or rural environment, and whether they have children (Espinal and Zhao 2015). For example, due to the rapidly and frequently changing economies, urbanization, and political reforms in Latin America, urban poverty has become more common in the region. This form of poverty is populated largely by women, who work mostly "informal" jobs that lack environmental and occupational regulations or consistent health insurance (Wasserman 1999). Additionally, the recent and ongoing Zika epidemic in Latin America highlights the intersections of health, gender, and politics in the region, with increased calls for improved abortion access and general reproductive care in a deeply Catholic region, even as Pope Francis has permitted contraceptives in Zika-stricken areas due to the serious birth defects associated with the disease (Grant 2016). While several countries (e.g., Argentina, Chile, Mexico) have made specific health reforms to improve access to health care and overall quality of life, this has not greatly improved health in the region due to persistent poverty levels and gendered job stratification (Gideon 2007).

Increasing research focuses on gender, health, and society in Latin America due to the region's rich history and culture, intricate political undercurrents, and complex identity issues. However, many Caribbean islands with similar backgrounds are regularly overlooked. This volume considers Latin America to encompass the traditionally recognized nation-states of Central America, South America, and the Caribbean, but also includes the oft-overlooked "black Caribbean," or West Indies. The editors of this volume believe that those nation-states and dependencies with similar historical trajectories and Romance languages (Spanish, Portuguese, and French) should of course be included in larger discussions of Latin America and the Caribbean, as they are similarly rooted in the Latin American colonial project. Yet, as we know, there are many Latin Americans who speak none of these languages. As Gates (2011) notes, the term *Latin America* lumps together speakers of Romance languages, yet ignores the millions of speakers of other regional languages such as English, Dutch, and various creole languages. However, he continues, "it seemed to be the most suitable and economical term that we could agree on to refer to this huge and richly various set of societies, each with its own unique history of slavery, genetic admixture, and race relations" (4). For this volume, cultural cues and historical continuities are just as valuable as linguistic ties, with Jamaican and Guadeloupean lives being of equal import.

With increasing emphasis on the complex ways in which gender and health intersect in Latin America, this volume offers a more detailed look at how gender embodies health inequities in the region and how societal woes impact and constrain gendered bodies in public social spheres. To this end, the authors developed this multidisciplinary volume by soliciting cutting-edge contributions from both established and emerging scholars in the fields of anthropology, gender studies, political science, public health, and Latin American studies, among many others. The resultant volume is organized thematically in relation to each chapter's primary focus on gender, health, and/or larger societal issues with gendered bodies. Our hope is that readers can connect with the work and apply an intersectional lens to the physical, mental, and social well-being of the peoples of Latin America and the Caribbean. In chapter 1, Savloff focuses on a women's collective in Buenos Aires, Argentina and its political work to erase the false dichotomy of the "outside" and "inside" of prisons. The collective, called *YoNoFui*, works with formerly and currently incarcerated women to gain visibility for their rights and expose the institutional violence carried out by the state. Through the use of workshops, they transform not only their subjectivities but also reconfigure a market and a state that continuously works to both monitor and disenfranchise women. This chapter questions the ways the personal and the political are entrenched by exploring how state surveillance imbues itself in the most intimate spheres of women's lives. It also explores Raquel Gutierrez Aguilar's concept of *entre mujeres* as a political power aimed to redefine the way we think of self-determination and interdependence.

Chapters 2 and 3 both consider localized Latin American masculinities and sexual practices in relation to sex work, albeit with very different communities and foci. In chapter 2, Perez-Bonilla focuses specifically on Dominican male sex workers, particularly those who engage in sex with other men (MSM) while continuing to self-identify as heterosexuals or *bugarrones*. She explores the ways and reasons these men have been made *invisibilizados* ("invisibilized") in the Dominican society by asking them to share their experiences in the sex-work industry. In addition, she considers Connell's (1995) theory on masculinities and the *activo/pasivo* (dominant/submissive) model discussed by Almaguer (1993) and Lancaster (2002) to understand how these men perceive themselves in society and vice versa. It is through this lens that she scrutinizes how they embody, (re)produce or (de)construct the discourses around masculinities and the *activo/pasivo* model in the Dominican context. She ends with a rumination on the acts and/or representations MSM sex workers put up for their clients as a mechanism to keep a regular clientele. For the men in this case study, gendered bodies intersect with gendered economies and emotional labor through romance tourism.

Chapter 3 situates the heterosexual commercial sex trade and economies of desire in contemporary Quito, Ecuador within the theoretical framework of Latin American masculinities advanced by Ecuadorean anthropologist Xavier Andrade. With interstitial dispatches from the field, Shepard and Tyndal argue that commercial sex in Ecuador has become more than a business transaction between individuals. It is a form of gender-role socialization where the *chongo* (brothel), an operating space for heterosexual desire, reinforces notions of male dominance as well as the need for male sexual experience. Masculinities and sexualities are intrinsically tied together in Latin America, intersecting with both gender and race in identity formations that are constantly in flux. With multiple masculinities to choose from at any given moment, it is often left to the public sphere to determine what symbols of manhood may look like for an individual. These labels can change for many reasons, up to and including fatherhood, gender performance in homosocial spaces, periods of revolution and periods of peace, and the role played within sexual encounters. As men begin to challenge their traditional roles in the reproductive sphere and the rearing of children, women are taking center stage as they both take control of their bodies and help to determine what it means to be a man. Masculinities and sexualities are racialized, with meanings and acts from both pre-Columbian times and the period of colonization acting in conversation with contemporary patterns of behavior. Finally, as globalization and migration also play an integral role in the dominant conceptions of masculinity and the formation of sexual identities, the chapter concludes with a survey of several chongos marketed to and by specific intersectional and global identities, places where gendered bodies regularly become bodily capital.

In chapter 4, Garriga-López and Rodríguez-Díaz examine how gendered power structures shape people's experiences with the Zika virus in the unincorporated U.S. territory of Puerto Rico. The authors use Charles Rosenberg's theory of epidemics as a tripartite process of meaning making within history to look at how the Zika epidemic became a fulcrum for gendered social power in Puerto Rico. They also discuss how the Zika virus epidemic in the Puerto Rican archipelago points to colonialism, poverty, and gender inequities as the most important barriers to health on the islands. This Zika virus outbreak and the resultant stories told about it highlight the need to understand and comprehensively address the social determinants of health that produce and reproduce health inequities in Puerto Rican society. The authors' analysis shows these were critical determinants in the spread and management of Zika. Finally, these conditions make tangible the deep connections between Puerto Rico as a U.S. colony and neocolonial dynamics in Central and South America in relation to the United States.

In chapter 5, Shan-Estelle Brown discusses how the people of Guadeloupe, an overseas region of France located in the Caribbean, have a high prevalence of sickle cell disease, a genetic disease of malformed red blood cells that predominantly affects people of African and Mediterranean descent. Sickle cell disease causes intense pain and shortened lifespan for affected individuals, yet no symptoms for carriers of the sickle cell trait. In Guadeloupe, one in eight citizens is a carrier for sickle cell disease and one in 260 babies born each year in Guadeloupe has sickle cell disease. Using a framework of critical medical anthropology, the chapter finds Brown investigating how a disease like sickle cell disease becomes situated in social contexts. Diseases and medical procedures represent intersections of power, class, race, gender, and culture. Gender affects how people in Guadeloupe see (1) who gets sick, (2) whose responsibility it is to stay well, (3) who should discuss illness, (4) who can discuss his or her own illnesses and with whom, and (5) who seeks health care. In Guadeloupe, it falls upon women to uphold these responsibilities. Brown's research recognizes the social importance of women, particularly mothers, as the *poto mitan*, the pillar of the family unit; this cultural phenomenon was shaped by colonialism and slavery, when male slaves lacked agency over their own lives. Thus, the belief in Guadeloupe today is that men and women are equal genetic contributors to their children, but their influence upon their children's lives has different proportions and purposes. Respondents in one-on-one interviews expressed awareness of sickle cell disease but considered themselves socially distant and therefore unconcerned about it, unless someone in their most immediate social network of closest family and friends had the disease. This local interpretation of concern has implications for sickle cell interventions and outreach in the region.

For centuries, ritual uses of the ayahuasca vine have been retooled by indigenous peoples in the Amazon for healing, auguring events, hunting, and telepathic communication. In chapter 6, Marcus and Fotiou consider ayahuasca shamans, retreat centers, and ayahuasca-related psychotherapy as a growing "network" of mental health care in the Peruvian Amazon and a localized manifestation of the global desire for non-Western therapeutic forms. In its current most popular form, a hallucinogenic tea made from the vine and other plants, ayahuasca attracts a growing international clientele for its role as a powerful medicine. The emphasis on its salubrious effects by westerners has brought increased attention to ayahuasca ceremonies and associated plant-based healing as effective therapeutic processes for the treatment of mental health conditions, notably anxiety, depression, trauma, addiction rehabilitation, and protracted grief. A proliferation of ayahuasca healing centers nourishes the ongoing therapeutic pluralism present in urban and peri-urban spaces of Peru's Amazon. From the international therapeutic community comprised of Western-trained psychotherapists, traditional shamans, and neo-shamans has emerged an ongoing dialogue between Western psychology and Andean-Amazonian cosmology in which therapeutic forms converge and mutually influence how clients and practitioners perceive illness, wellness, and healing. While calls for culturally-sensitive, cost-effective mental health treatment by the global health community have often been responded to by top-down, biomedical approaches with disease-specific concerns, these approaches funnel resources into improving access to psychological and psychiatric services to communities, yet few public health programs promote the growth and sustainability of local approaches to mental wellness.

In 2011, Chandler Burr made history in the Andes by becoming the first openly gay man to legally adopt children from Colombia. In their documentary analysis, Shepard and Lerman Ginzburg investigate this groundbreaking case, noting that prospective parents in the international LGBTQ community were regularly forbidden from adopting Andean children. As prospective parents, they faced institutionalized and social constraints due to both gender and sexual orientation. Presently, the children in need of families may be marginalized as "special-needs" adoptions; such needs may include a wide range of health conditions, ranging from lazy eye to debilitating illnesses, as well as Andean cultural conditions tied to race, age, and sibling sets. Birth parents may not be able to take care of children with special needs, or they may be afraid of the potential stigma surrounding perceived parental culpability. Furthermore, fear of addressing the cultural changes Andean children may face can contribute to the reluctance to give children up for adoption, particularly to LGBTQ parents. In chapter 7, we consider the positives and negatives of the international adoption process of Andean children with special needs and consider changes favorable to both potential LGBTQ parents and the Andean children in need of loving homes.

For chapter 8, Simpkins explores the lived experience of Black trans women within the Caribbean nation of Jamaica. Despite its marginal location and queer identity, the LGBTQI world movement is fused with pervasive intra-group marginalization along the lines of race, national identity, class, ableism, and, in many cases, gender performativity. These intersectional disjunctures work to present LGBTQI concerns as consensus issues (Cohen 1999), while the lives of its Black members, more specifically Black trans women, are made invisible and assumed to be disposable. As queer persons with citizenship in Western nations are fighting for marriage equality, Black trans women of Jamaica are fighting to stay alive and simultaneously come to represent a type of cross-cutting politics within the discourse of LGBTQI rights, health, and jurisprudence. Drawing on an analysis of law, newspapers, eye-witness accounts, and existing scholarship, this chapter places Black trans women at its center to illustrate the multifaceted impact of what Adrienne Rich terms as "compulsory heterosexuality."

Chapter 9 has Marcos et al. discussing the mental health impacts of gender-based violence as well as the resilience and survival strategies of *mujerxs* from the Northern Triangle—Guatemala, El Salvador, and Honduras—as they travel through Mexico. Contemporary flows of forced migration from the Northern Triangle are a result of push factors including gang violence, domestic violence, and other forms of gender-based violence. Particularly, cases of gender-based violence are often under-reported and unrecognized, and governments of these nations have both perpetrated this violence and failed to protect mujerxs from it. Notably, the United States' interventionist policies and actions have also contributed to the manifestation of violence. Accumulatively, this context has resulted in mental health impacts including the intergenerational transmission of trauma and layered traumas faced by mujerxs who are forced to migrate for their survival. In their transit through Mexico, forced migrants further face violence and are exploited by criminal networks (i.e., coyotes, cartels, trafficking, and extortion). In response, forced migrants continue to find alternative routes and create social networks of support. Rather than providing comprehensive trauma-informed aid, Mexico and the United States have responded to forced migration with the punitive measures of detention and deportation. In the case studies included in this chapter, we see that physical, mental, and social well-being are regularly impugned by global forces.

Transgender people have suffered various forms of prejudice and violence in Brazilian society. That violence and discrimination manifests at both the social and institutional levels. In the public sphere, this discrimination means non-recognition as subjects of law and, consequently, lack of access to constitutional rights, as in the case of integral health care. Chapter 10 notes that although Brazil has developed a few health policies for this population, they come from normative and hetero-centered conceptions, making transvestite and transsexual experiences and their demands invisible and illegitimate in public policy programs. Using empirical data about the transgender female reality in Brazil, Prado et al. aim to analyze their health conditions and their access to public services, as well as highlight the strategies they use to overcome barriers and broaden the debate on transgender access to public health. In Belo Horizonte, Brazil, they consider the health conditions of transvestite and transsexual sex workers and their (lack of) access to health services, which pushes the population to seek illegal and/or private health services for performing body changes and/or to practice self-medication. The authors also found a high rate of diagnosis of health problems in the population, creating great concern about both the indiscriminate use of hormonal drugs and HIV prevalence that is above the estimate of the general population. Finally, they note that access to the National Health System is reduced due to the transphobia that is expressed in this environment and the lack of programs that consider trans specificities. These factors only reiterate the sense of non-belonging, which contributes to the population's distance from these services, and the maintenance of stigmatized positions and inequalities in access to the National Health System.

The contributions for this volume walk readers through the various ways in which gender and health intersect both with each other and with structural factors, such as sexism, intimate-partner violence, racism, and other forms of marginalization in Latin America and the Caribbean (LAC). The various case studies presented in these chapters highlight the heterogeneity of gender and sexual identities in LAC, as well as the structural factors that shape these identities and the associated health outcomes. They emphasize both the intricacies of conducting research in this field and the imperativeness of the research in order to bring others' suffering to light and therein be a call to action to protect the very vulnerable populations being researched. Ultimately, as the contributors show, health is a shared obligation: at once an instrumental element for living well and a factor shaped by and for sociopolitical changes in the Latin American and Caribbean milieus. Gender differences in health outcomes persist to this day due to, for example, power struggles, multiple forms of violence, shifting political climates, and access to various resources. The contributors' groundbreaking work highlights the pressing need for more research, high-level policy change, and practical, hit-the-ground-running work that protects vulnerable members of society.

WORKS CITED

Baker, Peter and Tim Shand. "Men's health: time for a new approach to policy and practice?" *Journal of Global Health* 7, no. 1 (2017): 010306.

Cantú, Lionel. "Mexican Immigrant Men's Family Experiences." In *Perspectives on Las Américas*, edited by Matthew Gutmann, 245–273. Malden: Blackwell Publishing, 2003.

Espinal, Rosario and Shanyang Zhao. "Gender Gaps in Civic and Political Participation in Latin America." *Latin American Politics and Society* 57, no. 1 (2015): 123–138.

Frisco, Michelle L., Susana Quiros, and Jennifer Van Hook. "One Size May Not Fit All: How Obesity Among Mexican-Origin Youth Varies by Generation, Gender, and Age." *Demography* 53, no. 6. (2016): 2031–2043.

Gates, Jr. Henry L. *Black in Latin America.* New York: New York University Press, 2011.

Gideon, Jasmine. "Excluded from Health? Informal Workers' Access to Health Care in Chile." *Bulletin of Latin American Research: Journal of the Society for Latin American Studies* 26, no. 2 (2007): 238–255.

Grant, Melissa S. "Zika Virus Alters Catholic Church Policy on Contraception?" *Huffington Post*, February 25, 2016. https://www.huffingtonpost.com/melissa-s-grant/zika-virus-alters-catholic-church-policy-on-contraception_b_9301410.html. Updated December 6, 2017.

Martinez, Omar, Ji Hyun Lee, Frank Bandiera, E. Karina Santamaria, Ethan C. Levine, and Don Operario. "Sexual and Behavioral Health Disparities among

Sexual Minority Hispanics/Latinos: Findings from the National Health and Nutrition Examination Survey, 2001–2014." *American Journal of Preventive Medicine* 53, no. 2 (2017): 225–231.

Vlassof, Carol. "Gender Differences in Determinants and Consequences of Health and Illness." *Journal of Health, Population and Nutrition* 25, no. 1 (2007): 47–61.

Wasserman, Ellen. "Environment, Health, and Gender in Latin America: Trends and Research Issues." *Environmental Research* 80, no. 3 (1999): 253–273.

Chapter One

Freedom in Practice

Art Making and the Politics of Women's Incarceration in Argentina

Leyla Savloff

Life after prison can bring about as much uncertainty and as many hurdles as one would expect. Incarceration is a life-altering experience not only for the women doing time but also for their families and communities. Depriving women of their freedom creates ripple effects on a personal, collective, and structural dimension. Such effects are not undone when women are released from prison, but rather are waiting on the outside to be confronted.

"One of the striking paradoxes of the bourgeois ideological tradition," writes Angela Davis, "resides in an enduring philosophical emphasis on the idea of freedom alongside an equally pervasive failure to acknowledge the denial of freedom to entire categories of real, social human beings" (Davis 1998, 53). Denial of freedom, undoubtedly, calls for a consideration of what becomes possible and sayable in the struggle for a new subjectivity under the conditions of an ever-growing, profit-driven carceral state. As women in Argentina transition incarceration and later, their "release" to freedom, they organize and fight against institutional violence. The ways women reimagine themselves and their lives after enduring incarceration are the focus of this chapter.

For the past three decades, Latin America has been characterized by an increasing number of women facing incarceration (see Corda 2010). According to Luciana Boiteux, a feminist expert on drug policies, by 2037 women in Latin America will be represented more in prison than in positions of power (Boiteux 2017). *YoNoFui* is a women's collective in Buenos Aires, Argentina that works to thwart such disquieting statistics through community-based approaches and grassroots efforts. YoNoFui translates to It Wasn't Me, which is a humorous play on a common and ridiculed claim in prison. This collective works with women that have been involved in the criminal justice system and have experiences of incarceration, house arrest, or probation. They offer art-related workshops in women's prisons and in the collective's gathering space in Buenos Aires.

In this chapter, I explore the ways women in Buenos Aires forge new political selves that contest the oppressive forces of the carceral state. Specifically, it is concerned with expressions of subjective power that occur across multiple dimensions: at a personal level women alter what appear as inexorable destinies; at a communal level, women create bonds that strengthen their collective power and identity; and at a structural level, women organize to contest legal reforms that constrict the social life of prisons. I examine a journalism workshop offered outside of prison, a photography workshop offered inside the women's prison of Ezeiza, and the activism that YoNoFui engaged in during the time of my fieldwork. My analysis also addresses how recent political interventions in the Argentine criminal justice system create new challenges for women not only because they reduce access to education in prison, but also because they undermine the potentials of collective power engendered by collectives such as YoNoFui.[1]

Throughout this chapter, I conceive of the writing and art-making practices at YoNoFui as ways of becoming as well as expressions of collective power. The notion of becoming, as it has been recently theorized by João Biehl and Peter Locke, "emphasizes the plastic power of people and the intricate problematics on how to live alongside, through, and despite the profoundly constraining effects of social, structural, and material forces, which are themselves plastic. Unfinishedness is both a precondition and a product of becoming . . . a feature as generative to art and knowledge production as it is to living." (Biehl and Locke 2017, x). Such a generative feature emphasizes that freedom, in this context, is a process of becoming and is enacted through the daily practices of art making and activism.

In the space YoNoFui has in the city, there is a sign that reads "There is no body search that can see my soul." This was written by a participant of the poetry workshop in the women's prison and it reflects how freedom is enacted at YoNoFui. Raquel Gutierrez Aguilar (mathematician, philosopher, sociologist, and activist) warns us not to think of freedom as a lack of ties or an inexhaustible spectrum of possibilities (Gutierrez Aguilar 2015). Feminist accounts of freedom are not devoid of relationships to others, nor are they unaffected by structural and external impediments. Freedom can also be conceived, as philosopher Virginia Held suggests, as a practice aimed at inner processes of the self:

> the self-development of women involves changing the affective tastes, the emotional coloration, with which we experience the world, not only the outer obstacles in that experience. (Held in Deveux 1996, 224)

Shifting the attention to the inner workings of freedom does not mean that the structural forces that impinge on freedom are left unattended. Along with the sign mentioned above, there are other signs, photos, and a variety of cultural productions at YoNoFui that aim precisely at challenging state violence while strengthening the potential changes and growth made available by collective endeavors.

YoNoFui accompanies women's journeys as they transition between inside and outside the prison: as a collective, it supports artistic spaces and self-managed work; and through a critical reading of relations of power and existing structural inequalities, it seeks social transformation, the creation of new forms of engagements, and the constructions of solidarity.

I joined YoNoFui in February 2014 as a member of the "Social Support" team in a volunteer (unpaid) position. The Social Support team was involved, for example, in helping someone find an apartment, guiding them through the bureaucratic process of public assistance, finding a therapist, discussing their legal cases, and mostly, listening to them. Since YoNoFui is also considered a women's collective, my ethnographic fieldwork, carried out from February 2014 to March 2017, contextualized the potential contributions of such spaces as well as the possible becomings of feminist political power. As a member of the collective, I was expected to attend monthly *asambleas* and to participate in YoNoFui's social activism. Most importantly, the position required me to attend the workshops offered at YoNoFui, and hence interact daily with women staff and participants. I familiarized myself with handmade objects, recycled materials, pedagogical practices for formerly incarcerated individuals, and the daily struggles of women trying to reimagine their lives after leaving the repressive apparatus of the criminal justice system. This reimagining involved cultural productions and activism expressing something resembling freedom and desire.

During this time, freedom for the collective unfolded as a struggle and an exhausting practice. Activism, teaching in prison, public scholarship, art exhibits, and all the ways women make their work visible proved to be an arduous process. For many, coming out of prison is a frightening experience: stigmatization and lack of resources on the outside can offer an even less supportive environment than the prison setting. In Argentina, incarcerated women are usually part of impoverished communities, victims of several forms of abuse, and minor actors in the drug-traffic industry. As women are released from prison, most can only go back to the same precarious life they had before being detained, with the now-aggravating condition of a criminal record. In the face of such hardships, the cultural production and art-making practices of this women's collective opened up new paths of inquiry in which debating and redefining societal expectations for formerly incarcerated women becomes possible.

Feminist forms of political practice can reshape consciousness as well as the social fabrics of this capitalist world towards other more inclusive worlds. For example, one of the workshops offered inside the women's prison is on carpentry. While initially some women might be skeptical about this trade, it soon became an embodiment of everything that is possible through self-determination. In the carpentry workshop incarcerated women built a mobile bookshelf, repaired the playground in the visitors' area, and built children's tables and chairs to sell through the collective. Through this work, they re-defined not only their capabilities but also their environment. Women forged new selves (as carpenters, poets, photographers, workers) as they grappled with the oppressive consequences of confinement and the trauma of institutional violence. As women sought practices that enabled freedom, they engaged in a politics of becoming that altered the structural forces at play.

COLLECTIVE ENDEAVORS

"Without community, there is no liberation," writes the poet and activist Audre Lorde, adding that "poetry is not a luxury. It is a vital necessity of our existence." Poetry, affirms Lorde, is how we name the nameless: "It forms the quality of the light within which we predicate our hopes and dreams toward survival and change, first made into language, then into idea, then into more tangible action." (2007 [1984], 37, 112). While YoNoFui strived to create a community for liberation, their work revealed the multiple dimensions of becoming that are required in their efforts to end the gendered and institutional violence to which incarcerated women in Argentina are subjected. Such becomings not only illuminate the ways freedom is enacted as a practice, they also foreground the work of creativity that women accomplished in order to contest the constrictive forces of the carceral state.

YoNoFui began in 2002 as a poetry workshop in the women's prison of Ezeiza in Buenos Aires, Argentina. From the outset it was thought of not so much as a pedagogical space, where people from "outside" would teach to those "inside," but rather, it aimed to be a space of communion, where women came together to create and envision fertile futures for themselves and their families. The idea behind this project of encounters consisted of allowing freedoms to be expressed in manners that they had not been before, and which invited its participants to think of themselves in new ways.

YoNoFui aims to provide a visible and tangible connection between lives on the inside and the outside. For example, every year YoNoFui organizes poetry readings outside the penitentiary at cultural centers and in their space in Buenos Aires. Incarcerated women are able to attend these events by requesting special permits approved by the judges assigned to their cases. Poets are also invited to guest-lecture at the women's prison to strengthen the bridges and connections to worlds outside of prison. This dynamic, of coming out and inviting in, introduced and connected people that never would have met otherwise. Cultural events that include incarcerated women are spaces that support the formation of communal bonds between those incarcerated and those on the outside. These bonds are crucial in preventing women from going back to prison after they are released.

One other characteristic of this women's collective is that it includes people that have been incarcerated and others that have not. The purpose is to encounter one another and bridge the gap of what is considered outside and inside. The poetry workshop, for instance, involved a close-knit group of women that continued to meet after their release. The main concern recently released women brought up was the ability to work and earn an income. It was in these meetings that it was decided to expand the workshops to the "outside." As such, the workshops offered on the outside were conceived to support women's transitions. Their aim was to inspire self-management practices for careers that allowed them to work from home and on their own schedule.

In addition to the workshops, YoNoFui sells the products that they create in the workshops, such as clothing, notebooks, their magazine *YoSoy*, and carpentry items, as an effort to become a self-sustainable collective. The first additional workshop offered on the outside was textile design. At the time, all women's prisons in Argentina offered textile workshops so this served as the common denominator. One other important element of the workshops is that they are always led by pairs. By having two people facilitate a workshop there is always a sense of support, somebody else that is always there to help tackle the varying issues that may arise. When discussing certain topics that might be triggering, or if a debate turns heated, there is always someone available to go for a walk, and the workshop can continue with the work.

YoNoFui grew into a non-profit civic association that offered a variety of art-related workshops until finally reaching its current status as a worker cooperative. As Lorde writes, community is key for liberation, and YoNoFui offers a communal space where writing poetry is one of the ways women can begin to enact their future visions and impact their living conditions. Writing and art making emerge as processes of becoming that empower incarcerated women and their families, while also strengthening the social fabrics of the community at large. However, as women move away from the dehumanizing practices of prison life, these becomings towards freedom prove to be no easy feat. Freedom and struggle are always reworked in this process and writing and art making help illuminate the ways having a community and a safe space to come together can provide sustenance and form networks of support that were not always there.

My ethnographic analysis highlights freedom not so much as a fixed idea, but as a practice, assuming different meanings depending on the individual who enacts it. Writing is a practice of freedom. Working to redefine social roles is also a practice of freedom. Expressing your identity outside the heteronormative framework of sexuality can be a practice of freedom, as I will describe in Paula's story. The efforts carried out by the collective YoNoFui that are part of this analysis involve writing in the journalism workshop, taking photographs while in prison, and engaging in social activism to impact law reforms on incarceration issues. These examples contextualize how enacting freedoms is an exhausting and ongoing practice. At YoNoFui it involved, amongst other things, visiting government offices, writing press releases, calling in to radio shows, participating in panels, calling lawyers and social workers, applying for funding, teaching workshops, traveling back and forth to prisons (which are always so conveniently located in vexing locations), meeting with potential sponsors, volunteers, or partners, attending gatherings with other social organizations, protesting, creating media content to share on social media websites, constantly negotiating with the penitentiary system about what is allowed and what is possible in a workshop taught inside a prison, taking testimony about women's experiences inside the prison, the courts, and the public health-care system, and attending and providing testimony to congressional meetings where legislation concerning incarceration is being considered. YoNoFui relied on the assistance of volunteers, state funding from the Ministry of Education and the Ministry of Social Development, and contributions from friends and acquaintances who were lawyers, social workers, psychologists, artists, and entrepreneurs. Enacting freedom, in YoNoFui's case, involves a constant process of becoming.

WRITING AS A WAY OF BECOMING

The journalism workshop meets once a week, on Thursdays, on the outside. YoNoFui has its headquarters in the neighborhood of Palermo in central Buenos Aires. At the headquarters they held main events, meetings, sold their products, and offered some of their workshops, in particular book-binding, drawing, screen printing, and journalism. From the outside, the space has colorful walls decorated with graffiti murals and greenery. Inside, it is a loft-like space, with white-washed exposed brick. It is as vibrant as it is cluttered with the stuff that's been made, the products that they sell, and the stuff of making. There is usually a black cat named Luna in the space, and women meet surrounding a table. Luna, the eternally pregnant cat, had litters several times while I was there. While there was an invested interest in spaying her, Luna always managed to avoid getting placed in a crate, allegorically holding on to her own version of freedom.

On any given week, there might be between five and twenty women attending a workshop. As women arrive, there is always someone preparing *mate,* a traditional infused drink, and putting some snacks together. If weather permits, they might take the workshop outside. On the inside walls, you can find posters advocating for prison abolition, photography from the women's prisons, or pictures claiming justice for women that were murdered while incarcerated. The journalism workshop starts at 11 a.m. and the first half hour is spent catching up and waiting for everybody to arrive. Usually before noon, slowly, a certain order is manifested, and women begin their work. This work can involve reading book excerpts or newspaper articles and then writing in response to a prompt. Sometimes participants write a press release together, prepare questions for an interview, plan their messages for a women's march, or work on the content for their magazine *YoSoy*. On occasion there are guest lectures where writers, lawyers, artists, and other friends of YoNoFui come to share their knowledge. On a typical day at the workshop, women engage in reading critical texts and writing exercises. Their writing is then read out loud and women discuss their differing ideas. It is not always easy, particularly for a new participant, to read aloud texts that were just written and are often very personal. But with time, women get familiar with this process and begin sharing their work more often.

Paula is one of the most committed members of YoNoFui. She has been part of the collective for many years, attending the journalism workshop weekly. She wears short hair and prefers men's clothing. Even if people often refer to her as "Sir" and think she is going to the wrong restroom, it is important for her to be recognized as a woman. Paula positions her identity to disrupt hegemonic understandings of womanhood and challenge heteronormative assumptions of what women should look like. On this day, she was wearing a black beanie and took a deep breath before reading. Paula is a performer, amongst other things. She participated regularly in the theater of the oppressed and is an outspoken activist involved with a number of organizations. Nevertheless, she is always shy before reading her material. She has some childlike mannerisms, like opening up her chest with pride while smiling with shyness and looking down. She has a piercing in her eyebrow, and besides her beanie, she was also wearing several layers of clothes. It was winter, and even though the workshop meets between 11 a.m. and 2 p.m., the space was always cold. She hunched down to read and moved nervously. Grabbing the paper with shaky hands, she read:

> *It moves, the branch moves. Women's movement, empowered women. Extraordinary movement of dissidences. It moves. Smell of sauteed onion and mate lavado.*[2] *Texts with smell of scrambled ink. It moves with every heartbeat on the street. The drums and beat. It moves. We bring each other and distract each other. Movement of she-wolves. Explosive, furious movement. Movement and struggle. Disobedient voices, hoarse voices. The branch moves. If one yells, the world moves and all women respond. It moves and rage gets organized. We have arrived to disturb. We are the intruders. All the ones you've killed are today my muses. Hard voices, voices that do not quiet. Movement and struggle. We struggle for those who are not back. Here and elsewhere, up and down. We are the stone in your shoe, the ones keeping the score. We rebel against patriarchy. Brazen movement. Movement. Because we come out together, organized in unity.*

When the reading ends, Paula always tried to be serious, frowning her mouth for a few seconds until her face would blush and she couldn't hold her smile any longer, looking down but feeling proud. She apologized while beaming. I always wondered what part was her performance and what was her sweetness.

Paula's presence at YoNoFui was always relevant because she was never incarcerated nor involved with the criminal justice system. YoNoFui is not intended for incarcerated people only. It was always meant as a bridge, as a space of coming together. She was always outspoken about other prisons that are part of society. When she began attending the workshop, she had *problemas de consumo* as living on the streets often led her to abuse drugs and alcohol. According to her accounts (since this never happened while attending a workshop) she would also often get involved in violent situations as well as in aggressive behavior. Her presence allowed for the workshop to have meaningful conversations about belonging and the constructions of solidarity. When Paula got pregnant after being raped on the streets, she did not tell anyone. She was able to hide her pregnancy and one day she informed some members of the workshop that she was in the hospital and had given birth to a son. Due to a public policy put in place during the Kirchner Era, Paula was able to rent a room through public assistance in a tenement house turned hotel for her and her child, and her life as a transient person ended.[3]

During the time I knew her, I saw a lot of meaningful becomings in Paula's life: she committed to sobriety, secured stable income and housing, and got a handle on her anger management issues. From the first time I met her, Paula always liked to talk openly about her children. She told me about her daughter and her beautiful name and explained to me that after an open adoption process, her daughter lived with her co-parents. The story with her youngest son is longer and complicated, but he is now placed in an open adoption, as well. When we first met, her son was living in an orphanage close to YoNoFui and oftentimes she would visit the orphanage on her way to or from the workshop. She always thoroughly enjoyed spending time with the children present at YoNoFui and usually shared pictures of her children. Paula had a very playful personality, and it often seemed like she enjoyed children more than adults. She was always very aware and protective of the children present. In the heated debates and discussions that happened in the journalism workshop, it was always Paula that would remind us all that there were children in the space and we should watch our language and keep the dialogue amicable.

In her first years, Paula's involvement with YoNoFui was at times challenging. She often felt she did not belong and that she could not write about incarceration because she had never been "inside." She felt out of place, yet she kept coming back, week after week, because she understood that having a place that felt safe and stable was important for her life. While she received help in paying her rent from the government, that assistance was contingent on her living with her child. When she started the process of adoption for her son, her living situation immediately became more precarious. The stress of going back to the streets was overwhelming for Paula. Enacting freedom, in this case, was keeping a consistent routine and commitment to the collective. At the workshop, she engaged in using her own voice and her experiences in her writing. It was a process that involved a lot of work on her part as she learned to deal with the frustrations of the writing process. Attending the weekly workshop was not always easy. There was always *mate* and company. There was always a willingness to understand the other and a desire to build solidarity but considering the diversity of the women involved in the workshop, there were always disagreements, clashing personalities, and differing points of view.

When we read Virginie Despentes's *King Kong Theory*, a bold feminist memoir and manifesto, it sparked strong reactions. Paula liked the text, which is addressed to "the ugly ones: the old hags, the dykes, the frigid, the unfucked, the unfuckables, the neurotics, the psychos." The author, Despentes, writes:

> *In my case, prostitution was a crucial step in rebuilding myself after the rape. A business of dollar-by-dollar compensation, for what had been taken from me by brute force. I must have kept intact whatever I could sell to each client. If I could sell it ten times in a row, then it wasn't something that could be destroyed by use. My sex belonged to me only, it didn't lose value through being used, and it could be profitable. I was once again in an ultra-feminine position, but this time I was bringing in a profit.* (Despentes 2010 [2006], 67)

While the workshop usually focuses on Latin American authors and activists, participants often read texts such as Despentes's book that explore bountiful, controversial feminist questions that can be debated from diverse perspectives. Several older women in the workshop dismissed the idea that sex work could be liberating or empowering. Paula offered her insight into how you can be deprived of your freedom even if you are not in prison. And you can experience freedom in unpredictable places as well. You can be locked out on the outside by a bureaucratic system of public assistance that seems intent on excluding those in need. It was Paula's experience with the system on the outside that inspired her to become an activist. Paula wrote about her experiences living on the streets to emphasize that transient people are not all the same, that opportunities are worth giving, that safe spaces are important, and community building is key to practices of freedom.

PINHOLE PHOTOGRAPHY: ART AS A WAY OF BECOMING

In addition to creating a space for gathering, YoNoFui defends expressiveness whether it is through the written word, the products they create, activism, or through their photography workshop. The photography workshop is taught inside one of the women's prisons in Ezeiza, Buenos Aires. Below, I present photos taken by participants of YoNoFui. There are two elements about this photography workshop that are relevant to consider. One particularity of this women's prison in Buenos Aires is that it has a prison nursery. Prison nurseries are special prison units designed to keep mother and child together. In Argentina, over 80 percent of incarcerated women are mothers and women in prison can choose to keep their children with them until the age of four. The photography workshop included participants that were housed in the prison nursery. Hence, in some of the images created by this workshop, babies or elements and spaces related to child-rearing are present.

One other element to consider is that the photography workshop is taught using a special technique called "pinhole photography." Pinhole photography is lensless photography. It consists of a small box with a tiny hole that replaces the lens. Light passes through the hole and an image is formed in the camera. Pinhole cameras are small or large, improvised or designed with great care. Cameras have been made of seashells, oatmeal boxes, soda cans or cookie containers. A pinhole camera is simply a box, with a tiny hole on one side, and film or photographic paper on the opposite side. A camera used with the pinhole method can be made with empty matchstick boxes, like the ones used by YoNoFui, which are safe for prison due to their unthreatening character.

Correctional institutions often blur distinctions between "benefits" and "rights" and the women's prison of Ezeiza was no exception. Visitations, proper nutrition, access to health care and education, being able to shower—these were all things that could be easily taken away for a variety of reasons. Taking a class in prison was no different. It required vast amounts of effort and insistence, as the penitentiary operated with plenty of paperwork moving at a snail's pace. Class materials were heavily inspected and sanctioned. The long commute was hard for those teaching when often students did not show up. These absences were explained, more often than not, by guards who had "forgotten" to go and get students for their classes. Other times, prison guards were late. Arbitrarily, the penitentiary could cancel daily activities without warning.

Educational spaces are disappearing in prisons and classes like this one are rare. In 2014, a photo exhibit called *Iluminaciones* showcased the work that emerged from the photography workshop. The premise of the workshop was to promote self-expression, to see the space they occupied from different viewpoints and in turn, think of themselves from a different perspective. Because pinhole photography takes a few minutes to capture an image, the time of image-making was meant for introspection. "Pinhole cameras invite a reflection of the moment," said the class facilitator, Gabriela. "Because they take time, we can only take a few photos each class. This calls for a more critical view on what the image will actually show" (*YoSoy*, no. 2, 2016).

What begins as a class that a woman takes to get out of her unit for a while, a class that uses a camera made out of a matchstick box, allows for women, months and years later, to then stand in a photo exhibit as an artist, able to

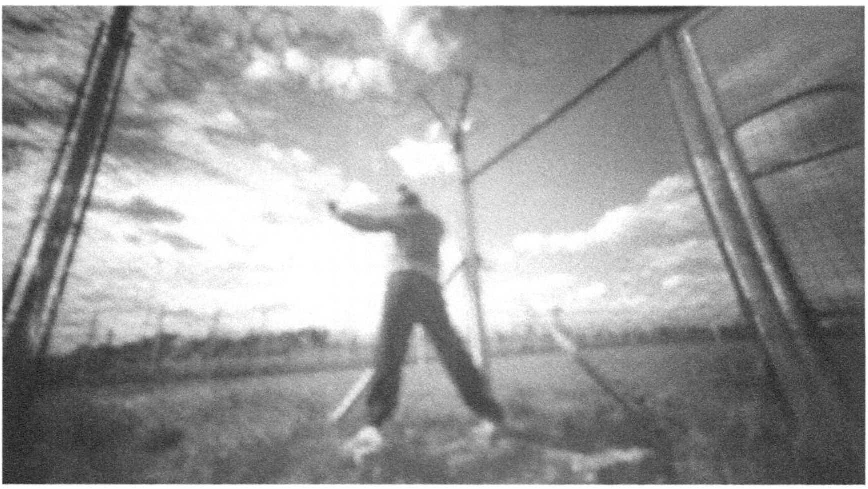

Figure 1.1.
From *Iluminaciones*, courtesy of YoNoFui

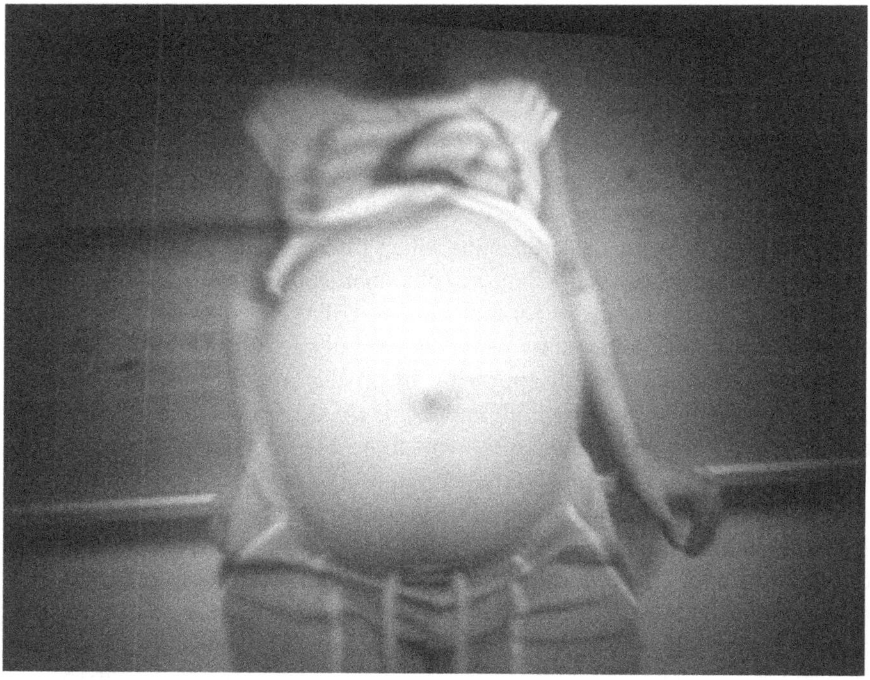

Figure 1.2.
From *Iluminaciones,* courtesy of YoNoFui

discuss her work and talk about herself in a different way. To imagine herself from another viewpoint: as a maker of images, as someone that is proactive in her life and deliberate in her expression, that has talent to share and that is able to express artistically. She becomes part of a meaning-making process and contributes to cultural productions that are worth looking at.

Regarding her experience in the photography workshop, Soledad, a member of YoNoFui, stated, "Even if the end result was uncertain, it was a space during the deprivation of my freedom that allowed me to make decisions, to have control over certain processes" (*YoSoy*, no. 2, 2016). While the prison setting strains opportunities to express oneself in artistic ways, both the poetry workshop and the photography workshop provide a platform where communication and projecting oneself as writers and artists become possible. Carmen, another workshop participant, noted that "when I take a picture, I look for the same thing as when I write: to translate an emotion, a heap of sensations from a specific moment . . . what seems inexplicable with words" (*YoSoy*, no. 2, 2016). Further, in a prison setting where time moves at a particular pace and rhythm, somewhat fixed and structured, the photography workshop provides the alternative to imagine life otherwise—"photography

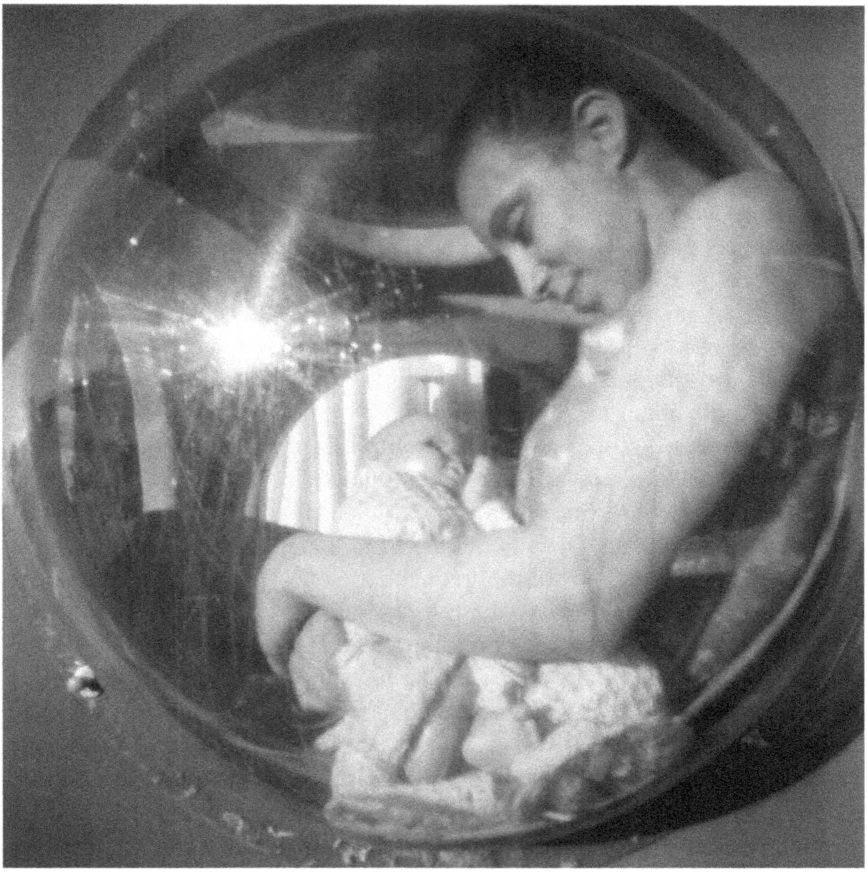

Figure 1.3.
From *Iluminaciones,* courtesy of YoNoFui

gave me the possibility of reinventing my days, of reinventing the same patio," adds Carmen.

The photography workshop is more than anything a space for gathering, for using the senses in a collective way, and for reflecting about emancipatory practices and alternatives to incarceration. In his essay, "Literature and Life," Giles Deleuze writes:

> Even when it is a woman who is becoming, she has to become-woman and this becoming has nothing to do with a state she could claim as her own. . . . To become is . . . to find a zone of proximity, indiscernibility, or indifferentiation . . . where one could no longer be distinguished as *a* woman, *an* animal, or *a* molecule—neither imprecise nor general, but unforeseen and nonpreexistent, singularized out of a population rather than determined in a form. (1998, 1)

Iluminaciones, the name of the photo exhibit, allows us to see how participating in a photography class in prison can lead to a photo exhibit in an art gallery. It involves a process of becoming, of strengthening a collective identity as well as an individual one, that seeks to promote change in the social life of prisons, to find a zone of proximity, as Deleuze expressed. When women gather around the camera to plan each photo they take, the photography workshop provides the platform to create strategies of personal and social becomings, since it involves a collective construction of the gaze. As described by the class facilitator Gabriela, "these are not denouncement photos, but an attempt to capture the everyday lives of women deprived of freedom; they show the quotidian efforts women engage in to live, to mother inside prison walls, to build a space of light that allows them to resist and from there think about new possibilities."

Expressiveness is fostered in all YoNoFui's workshops not only amongst the women themselves but amongst the organization as well. For example, the textile design workshop often has participants confined to house arrest interested in learning a skill and working from home with a sewing machine. One afternoon while in YoNoFui, I remember one of the "facilitators"[4] of the workshop noticed that some of the pillows sewn by a woman under house arrest had an added accessory, a pom-pom attached to the zipper that solved a number of issues: it did away with the potential discomfort of the zipper and it eased the process of opening the cover of the pillow so that it could be removed for washing. This was used as a teaching moment and it was also decided that from that moment on, pillows will come with pom-poms. Allowing different women to do their work from home opened up the possibilities in which creative expressions became possible through the work, invigorating moments of inventiveness that improved the product as well as strengthened the organization.

ACTIVISM AGAINST INSTITUTIONAL VIOLENCE

YoNoFui fosters community building through the workshops they offer and through the activist work in which they engage. While the collective often hosted cultural events such as poetry readings and festivals, they also participated in protests related to gender and institutional violence. YoNoFui designed and produced a big flag with their name "YoNoFui—organización política y social," and the borrowed phrase "the only thing unreal is the fence." The phrase gracing the flag is from a poem by Paco Urondo (1930–1976), a controversial figure who stood against state violence. He was also a writer and journalist and was assassinated by the Argentine Security Forces during the last military dictatorship. An excerpt from the poem, written while he was detained in a prison in Buenos Aires reads:

> On the other side of the fence is the reality, on
> this side of the fence there is also
> reality; the only thing unreal is the fence.[5]
>
> Paco Urondo, Prison of Villa Devoto, April 1973

YoNoFui's flag includes the phrase, "The only thing unreal is the fence" because part of their work is to challenge the prison system and make visible its institutional violence. According to one of the founders, Elena, their goal is not to "make prison better," but to support women after incarceration. This involves engaging in activist practices and bureaucratic and legal procedures to improve the living conditions of women, both inside and outside of prisons. During 2014–2017, part of this political work involved contesting the reforms of the federal law 24.660. This law details the specific ways in which deprivation of freedom should be carried out by the state: how individuals should be treated while incarcerated, the disciplinarian methods involved, the rewards, access to work, education, health care, spirituality, social and family relations, and social assistance after prison.

YoNoFui contested these reforms which they considered regressive as they involved harsher sentencing, reduction of parole (mandating to serve the full sentence instead), cuts in the daily leaves that are allowed once release date approaches, and almost no access to education. In 2016, the penitentiary decided that no cameras were allowed in the photography class, so YoNoFui had to resort to offering a theoretical photography class. From that class emerged the photo exhibit *Imagenes Guardadas*, which displays written descriptions of imagined photos, and the photos that other women took on the outside, based on the descriptions. The exhibit was hosted at the Matienzo cultural center, in the neighborhood of Almagro, Buenos Aires, and it was successful in both strengthening the links between the inside and the outside and making visible the impacts that institutional violence has on educational spaces.

The law reforms in question seek to reduce not only educational opportunities (currently available to only 3 percent of incarcerated individuals), but health-care benefits and work opportunities, as well. The reform switched the language to emphasize work, health care, and education as "benefits" rather than rights. These benefits are left to the discretion of the penitentiary to decide which inmates, if any, can receive them. Further, the reform does not consider nor suggest the implementation of policies (such as work quotas) to address the discrimination individuals with criminal records face once they are released. Work prospects for formerly incarcerated individuals, especially when they cannot invest their time while incarcerated in education or work experience, become slim to none. Such hurdles become harder for women who are often single heads of households, solely in charge of child care.

Concomitantly, this reform endorses the penitentiary as the sole power in charge of incarcerated lives since it greatly reduces the participation of outside professionals (offering classes, workshops, or other type of "benefits"). Professionals that work outside the penitentiary are critical in making the transition to a life away from prison possible. Before the reform, the judicial power was in charge of handling those in parole, conditional, or any other alternative in sentence completion (such as house arrest). With the new modifications, the penitentiary system alone will be in charge of the entirety of the sentence. Lawmakers appealed to "closing the revolving door" to justify the reduction in alternatives to incarceration. "Closing the revolving door" also means reducing access to education and the connections to social organizations and universities, therefore diminishing the permeability between the outside and the inside. Without incentives for education, the prison will in fact turn into a much more closed system overseen and controlled by the penitentiary alone. The penitentiary system in Argentina is infamous for obliterating prisoner's rights, for torturing prisoners, and for allowing "suicides" to happen on a regular basis. In November 2016, the Observatory Against Gender Violence (OVG) in Buenos Aires denounced violent searches at the women's prison of Los Hornos on the night of November 26 (Calotti 2016). That night, prison guards destroyed women's property, transferred five women to another prison, and placed several others in solitary confinement. The next day, there was a scheduled event to celebrate students ending the academic year with several university professors in attendance. The event did not take place and the women were punished. This example is one of the many that are routinely executed in prison settings. Granting more power and less control checks to such a system can only worsen living conditions inside the prison walls.

This law reform directly affects the work of YoNoFui as they will no longer be able to offer their workshops in the women's prison. Learning a trade, or acquiring a high school degree (or elementary school degree) will no longer be possible goals to pursue while incarcerated.

Carmen, a member of YoNoFui, testified against the reform, letting legislators know that she came to know YoNoFui as an incarcerated woman. She spent eight years behind bars, and during that time she came in contact with the workshops offered by YoNoFui, specifically, the photography and poetry workshops. She declared that it is through her participation in those workshops that today she can have a life where her writing and her voice matter. She also testified that while she was incarcerated the workshops were the only spaces where she could feel like a person. After participating in the workshops, she was able to fund her *editorial cartonera*, a press that publishes books using cardboard and recycled materials. During her testimony, she stressed that while she was the founder, this was a collective effort in which her classmates assisted and supported her to make this project happen. As Lorde describes, "Interdependency between women is the only way to the freedom which allows the I and 'be,' not in order to be used, but in order to be creative" (Lorde 1984, 111). This interdependency of acknowledged and equal difference is what generates the power to imagine and create other ways of being in the world, such as a women's collective like YoNoFui.

The reforms to constrict the social life of prisons come on the heels of a highly repressive and punitive discourse that correlates with the expansion of neoliberal policies. This was not always the case, as historian Lila Caimari recounts in *Apenas un Delincuente. Crimen, castigo y cultura en la Argentina 1880–1995.* In her historical analysis, Caimari describes how, beginning in the late 1800s and growing into the 1930s, an imaginarium of the convicted as an individual worthy of compassion coupled with a thorough depiction of the prison setting as rampant with plentiful forms of abuse, convinced the public discourse that the punitive experience of the carceral setting was utterly ineffective (Caimari 2012). The advent of dictatorships that plagued Argentina and the advancement of capitalism, slowly but steadily dissolved the humanization of those incarcerated, or, for that matter, any sense of communal bonds. As Diana Taylor describes it, "Just as human beings disappeared, so did civil society" (Taylor 1997).

Anthropologist Rita Segato introduces the term "pedagogy of cruelty" to refer to the preying capitalist economic structures that require unmitigated individualism and the dissolution of communal bonds to sustain its power. The "pedagogy of cruelty" teaches us that relationships amongst objects are elevated from relationships of communal bonds, hence making empathy undesirable amongst community members. It affects our capacity to put ourselves in the shoes of the other, which is the condition for empathy, care, and respect. Our skin only gets thicker and mass media foments that morbid pulse (Segato 2016). Maria, one of the founding members of YoNoFui, wrote an article for a major newspaper stating how this reform violates the principle of resocialization, which is the only basis for conviction in the current Argentine Constitution (Medrano 2017). It also violates International Treaties to which Argentina has subscribed, worsening prison conditions by overcrowding, increasing health risks for prisoners, and intensifying the risk of violence and death. Reducing the daily exits and the benefits that accumulate as the release date approaches removes the motivation for those imprisoned to follow rules.

Standardizing how one spends time incarcerated means that it ceases to matter how one invests their time while in prison, presupposing that individual behavior does not count. Whether you study, work, learn a trade, have good conduct, or do absolutely nothing does not make a difference for the system. Sentencing is the same, regardless of your actions. The motivations and encouragement to avoid prison life and seek opportunities for work and/or education become a moot point as confinement becomes an inexorable destiny.

YoNoFui's trajectory inside and outside of prison affirms that education and work while in prison, as well as incentives such as daily exits, broadens the network of affective relationships and financial support. This network makes it possible for individuals to lead a life outside the prison system. The privileges that one accrues as one is about to be released prepare individuals to transition to life on the outside. It does this by making this progression a slow process, rather than an abrupt change.

If lawmakers want to address "the revolving door" and prevent recidivism, Medrano's article suggested two bills that are at stake to address employment opportunities after incarceration. One affects YoNoFui to the core as it pertains to allowing people with criminal records to be part of the administrative council of cooperatives. For YoNoFui, becoming a worker cooperative involved a lot of slow arduous labor. It was devastating to learn that some of its founders, because of their past convictions, could not occupy any official capacity within the cooperative that they themselves built. YoNoFui and other organizations working with formerly incarcerated people have been campaigning for the last few years to get this regulation modified. The other bill proposes to hold employers accountable for fulfilling work quotas for people with criminal records. Thus, rather than enforce harsher sentencing and aggravate prison conditions, a better alternative would be to generate public policies that ameliorate the conditions of life after prison. When discussing recidivism, the experience of freedom is one that should encompass social inclusion and employment opportunities to create feasible opportunities for those who regain their freedom.

FREEDOM AS STRUGGLE

The work of YoNoFui challenges the perception of the prison as a closed institution. "The only thing unreal is the fence" reads YoNoFui's flag. The collective demonstrates and insists that the prison is very much entrenched in society and there is a relevant continuum between the prison and civil society. Public policies that aim at "closing the revolving door" reduce educational opportunities in prison and the traffic of individuals from the outside. Offering opportunities such as spaces of education is a better alternative than empowering an already punitive and corrupt system. In the journalism workshop offered in the prison of Ezeiza, Silvia, one of the participants, wrote:

> Writing provokes spaces of reflection in which we can assimilate the different emotions that traverse us. Rage, anger, impotency and anguish translate onto the paper to become something else. And that mutation begets the possibility of processing that pain differently. That is also what our work is about: thinking of ourselves *with* others, finding ourselves in a text or in a poem, and thriving together.
>
> Why do I sometimes feel invisible?
>
> I want my life back, my freedom, my family and I only have one objective: "Behave well" but on this side, what does that mean?
>
> It means putting up with all the shit that comes my way, every injustice, every threat, I feel that as days go by, "behaving well" means I need to annul myself, minimize myself in this world where the loudest rules, it sucks. . . . Just to regain my freedom I have to be invisible. . . .

The prison system is designed to make people like Silvia feel the way she does. Interventions such as the ones YoNoFui offers, grant women the space to come together and expand their political imagination. This is not a job training program; it isn't a therapeutic exercise, either. Their work is presented as a tool to promote new practices for new social roles. In 2002, Maria Medrano decided to offer a poetry workshop in a women's prison, and slowly, YoNoFui began to take shape. Today, more than fifteen years later, the organization is supported by women's work and by contributions from other institutions (such as the Ministry of Labor, the Ministry of Social Development, and Universidad de Buenos Aires), small businesses, artists, and volunteers. Their objective is to make visible the particular needs that incarcerated women and their families have; to promote respect for human rights; and to strengthen the constitution of collective endeavors. Collective endeavors can bring about social transformation through their self-reflective action, their capacity for resistance, and by providing a discursive space where collaboration emerges from a critical and liberating perspective. Collective endeavors open up new critical spaces where collective strategies for individual and social transformation become possible.

This chapter has argued that expressions of subjective power that contest the oppressive forces of the carceral state are produced through collectives such as YoNoFui in Buenos Aires, Argentina. These are meaningful becomings of women transitioning out of prison life, who organize social events and protests, while also producing art together. My analysis addressed how recent political interventions in the Argentine criminal justice system create new challenges for women not only because they reduce access to education in prison, but also because they undermine the potentials of collective power engendered by collectives such as YoNoFui. Their writing and art-making practices redefine freedom as a process and a struggle that always needs reworking and is in a constant state of unfinishedness. In this case, enacting freedoms is an exhausting and ongoing practice. The collective, however, not only contributes with critical prison perspectives and feminist interventions to the criminal justice system but also as a source of social support. Collective endeavors such as YoNoFui provide a safe space for feminist practices to strengthen their social fabrics and politics.

NOTES

1. Except for Maria Medrano, founding member of the collective YoNoFui, and Luna, the cat, names and identifying features have been changed.
2. "Mate lavado" is a term that refers to the traditional infused drink of yerba mate after it has been watered down many times and hence has lost its flavor (washed mate).
3. The Kirchner Era refers to the presidencies of Nestor Kirchner (2003–2007) and Cristina Fernandez de Kirchner (2007–2015), which were characterized by human rights policies, nationalization of industries, and an emphasis on workers' rights, amongst other measures.
4. YoNoFui is a collective that works in a horizontal manner and the colloquial language often used in work environments many times failed. As mentioned previously, YoNoFui also tries to move away from a pedagogical framework. Hence, the term "teacher" is avoided.
5. Translation by the author.

WORKS CITED

Biehl, João and Peter Locke. 2017. "Foreword. Unfinished" in *Unfinished. The Anthropology of Becoming,* edited by João Biehl and Peter Locke. Duke University Press.

Boiteux, Luciana. 2017. "En los próximos 20 años vamos a estar más representadas en cárceles que en los espacios de poder" Interview by Viviana Escales. *LatFem*, September 22. Accessed September 17, 2018. http://latfem.org/en-los-proximos-20-anos-vamos-estar-mas-representadas-en-las-carceles-que-en-los-espacios-de-poder/.

Caimari, Lila. 2002. *Apenas un Delincuente. Crimen, castigo y cultura en la Argentina, 1880–1955.* Siglo XXI Editores Argentina.

Calotti, Gabriela. 2016. "Requisa violenta y suspensión de cierre de ciclo educativo en la cárcel de mujeres de Los Hornos" Contexto. November 26, 2016. Accessed December 11, 2018. https://www.diariocontexto.com.ar/2016/11/26/requisa-violenta-y-suspencion-de-cierre-de-ciclo-educativo-en-la-carcel-de-mujeres-de-los-hornos/?fbclid=IwAR16bx9iYwM9uJQPuQSu-oiZe3vykn5u5mUHrmgHFkEEhJyGT-BLeb03BHQg.

Corda, Raul Alejandro. 2010. Encarcelamientos por delitos relacionados con estupefacientes en Argentina. *Sistemas Sobrecargados. Leyes de drogas y cárceles en América Latina*. Transnational Institute. Electronic Document, accessed March 2, 2018. http://www.druglawreform.info/es/publicaciones/sistemas-sobrecargados.

Davis, Angela. (1998 [1969]). "Unfinished Lecture on Liberation—II." In *The Angela Y. Davis Reader*, edited by Joy James, 53. Blackwell Publishers.

Deleuze, Giles. 1998 [1993] "Literature and Life." In *Essays Critical and Clinical*, translated by Daniel W. Smith and Michael A. Greco. London: Verso.

Despentes, Virginie. 2010. *King Kong Theory*. The Feminist Press at CUNY.

Deveux, Monique. 1996. "Feminism and Empowerment: A Critical Reading of Foucault." In Susan J. Hekman *Feminist Interpretations of Michel Foucault*, 2118–238. Pennsylvania State University Press.

Geronimo, Alan. "Reforma Carcelaria: kirchnerismo y macrismo a favor del punitivismo." In *La Izquierda Diario*, July 6, 2017. Accessed March 2, 2018. https://www.laizquierdadiario.com/Reforma-carcelaria-kirchnerismo-y-macrismo-a-favor-del-punitivismo?id_rubrique=1201.

Gutiérrez Aguilar, Raquel. 2015. *Desandar El Laberinto. Introspección en la femineidad Contemporánea*. Buenos Aires: Tinta Limón.

Lorde, Audre.1984. *Sister Outsider: Essays and Speeches*. Berkeley: Crossing Press.

Medrano, Maria. 2017. "No en el nombre de Micaela." *Página/12*, April 21. Accessed March 2, 2018. https://www.pagina12.com.ar/32956-no-en-el-nombre-de-micaela?_ga=1.172425376.2006573869.1491754503.

Segato, Rita. 2016. *La Guerra Contra Las Mujeres*. Madrid: Traficantes de Sueños.

Taylor, Diana. 1997. *Disappearing Acts. Spectacles of Gender and Nationalism in Argentina's 'Dirty War.'* Duke University Press.

Tinta Revuelta. 2016. "Cuando El Tiempo De Espera Cambia Las Formas." In *YoSoy*, no. 2, 18–26.

Chapter Two

Dominican *Bugarrones*

(in)Visibility, Masculinities, and Same-Sex Performances

Lauren M. Pérez-Bonilla

SEX WORK IN THE DOMINICAN REPUBLIC

The Island of the Dominican Republic (henceforth "the Island") is known as a top destination for sex tourism (Fieser 2013), where foreigners go to enjoy its natural resources and fulfill their fantasies of dominating the Caribbean body. The United States Centers for Disease Control and Prevention defines sex tourism as "travel planned specifically for the purpose of [having] sex" (CDC 2013). With locals who offer these services at a reasonable rate that could mean a monetary transaction, or the exchange of material goods deemed as "valuable" (International Justice Mission 2015, 5). These locals are generally referred to as commercial sex workers (CSWs). As of November 2017, an estimated total of 25,000 people on the Island are said to be dedicated to sex work (Vargas 2017). As a result, the territory is globally positioned as the fourth country with the highest sex worker populations compared to their overall population.

This chapter focuses specifically on Dominican male sex workers, particularly those who engage in sex with other men (MSM) and identify themselves as heterosexuals or *bugarrones*, as they are commonly known on the Island. Unlike female or transsexual CSWs, there is not that much information available on male CSWs nor bugarrones. Consequently, I explore the ways and reasons these men have been made invisible or *invisibilizados* ("invisibilized") in the Dominican society by asking them to share some of their experiences in the sex work industry with me. *Invisibilización* (invisibilization) refers to a process of "systematically oppressing, suppressing and weakening the identity of [deviant social] groups as a mechanism [to preserve] cultural homogeneity" (Bastidas and Torrealba 2014, 517, 526). As a way to examine how bugarrones are made (in)visible, I rely on questions targeting media exposure, institutional aid and support, social stigma and discrimination, and mobility in public spaces when offering their services.

In addition, I explore Connell's (1995) theory on masculinities and the *activo/pasivo* (dominant/submissive) model discussed by Almaguer (1993) and Lancaster (2002), to understand how these men perceive themselves in society and vice versa. Inquiries regarding their roles as bugarrones versus the roles they perform within their regular sexual life were made. Together with that, questions focusing on emotional development towards their clients were also raised with these men. Through this, I intend to scrutinize how they embody, (re)produce or (de)construct the discourses around masculinities and the *activo/pasivo* model in the Dominican context.

As a third element, the present work focuses on same-sex performances based on the acts and/or representations MSM sex workers put up for their clients, as a mechanism to keep a regular clientele. Here, I turn to concepts such as Pruitt and LaFont's (1995) *romance tourism* (connections between tourists and locals based on feelings and emotions over physical/sexual acts) and Hochschild's (1983) emotional labor (the type of work that requires the worker to suppress or filter certain emotions in order to satisfy their customers). It is important to note that the word "performance" does not have a direct or literal translation in Spanish. Thus, I employed words such as *actuación* (act/acting) and *representación* (representation) when conducting the interview process with my subjects. The men in my sample agreed on using feelings as a tactic to increase their chances of earning more money from a steady, trustworthy source: a foreign gay man. Nevertheless, engaging in such dynamics seemed to push these men out of their comfort zone. They realized that, even though they get to treat their client as a lady (i.e., sweet-talking them), the customer is still a man. Consequently, it can be argued that, by engaging in same-sex sexual encounters, the men included in the study contest the ideology of the Dominican man.[1]

As most of the literature available on sex work(ers) in the Caribbean region focuses principally on female sex workers (Brennan 2004; Cohen 2006; Sanchez Taylor 2006; Compres 2009; Pardais 2017), the delimited hotelier/tourism sector (Cabezas 2009), and HIV/AIDS (Tabet, de Moya, Rosado Holmes, et al. 1996; Padilla, Castellanos, Guilamo-Ramos, et al. 2008; Pope, Hodge, Donastorg, et al. 2014), by focusing on the abovementioned areas (visibility, masculinities, and same-sex performances), the following work seeks to portray a more humane side of the topic. By concentrating on the area of *La Zona Colonial*—the historic center of Santo Domingo city—where CSWs are not policed as much as they are in tourist areas, and employing a qualitative methodology, I aim for an intersectional, multilayered approach to sex work, in order to stop depicting these people as hypersexual (Kempadoo 2004, 11) disease carriers from which one has to be protected. Through this approach, then, my goal is to include these men's voices in the overall conversation about sex work taking place at the moment. Subsequently, the addition of their experiences to academia will allow for a more significant and representative understanding and exploration of Caribbean, Latin American, and Latina/o sexualities.

METHODOLOGY

For this project I rely on different kinds of qualitative information-gathering methods which include (but are not limited to) participant observation, informal conversations, content analysis, archival data from governmental and non-governmental organizations (NGOs), and semi-structured interviews with male CSWs and institutional personnel. The use of semi-structured interviews in this study allowed me to verify to what extent the broader academic and policy literature is representative of Dominican male sex workers' realities. In order to protect my subjects from being identified in this study, fictional names are employed and pseudonyms (if any) were changed. The other data-gathering methods enabled me to build a comprehensive picture of the context in which sex work takes place globally and locally—specifically, by placing it as a contemporary and on-going issue within Dominican society. Although I spent considerable time collecting and constructing my literature review for this study, the primary empirical source for this chapter are the interviews with bugarrones.

The aforementioned techniques were employed during two different periods: from May to June 2017 ("exploratory phase") and December 2017 to January 2018 ("interviewing phase"), through which I carried out fieldwork in the Dominican Republic. In the first period, I identified and verified local institutions involved in the topic, as well as established contact with scholars and activists interested in both the subject and my project. During this initial phase, I familiarized myself with locations and spaces where sex work and *bugarronería* (or gay sexual activity) took place. Even though I spent plenty of time carrying out participant observation at La Zona Colonial and Boca Chica (the nearest beach town to Santo Domingo), I limit my analysis to the former for two reasons. The first is that it is a space in which locals have easy access compared to other touristy locations on the Island. Secondly, the fact that multiple gay discos and bars are located here made La Zona Colonial even more suitable for the present study. The rest of the summer was spent going back and forth to visit multiple nongovernmental organizations (NGOs) located around the capital city.

Moreover, I carried out content analysis of local newspapers and news outlets as a way to interpret the level of coverage that sex work(ers) receive in the local press. Daily newspapers including *Listín Diario*, *El Día*, *Diario Libre*, *Hoy*, and *El Caribe* were my periodicals of choice, as they have the widest circulation and are among the most popular on the Island. During the exploratory phase, I paid particular attention to concepts such as "sex work," "sex tourism," "tourism," "*chapeo,*" "prostitution," "prostitute(s)," "*bugarrones*," "sex worker(s)," "*prepagos* (pre-paids)," and "escorts." The word *chapeo* has become popular in the Dominican mainstream culture. By definition, it means to remove the weeds from the soil. In this specific context, however, it alludes to the act of a young woman cleaning out an older man's wallet by being seductive towards him. In a way, this could be seen as a sugar daddy–sugar baby relationship. Nonetheless, these men believe that they have other attributes that allow them to conquer the young ladies, at least until they run out of money. When that occurs, they realize they have been wiped clean or, more colloquially speaking, *chapeados*. Subsequently, another word related to sex work in the Dominican Republic—as well as in other parts of the Spanish-speaking Caribbean—is that of *prepago* (pre-paid). As the name indicates, these are people who get a payment before they engage in any sexual act with their client. *Prepagos* are very similar to escorts in the sense that many of them possess a good education and looks. Because of the massive migration of Venezuelans into the country, female CSWs are complaining as they appear to be taking clients away from them (Jimenez 2017). The public is attracted to Venezuelan women as their fees are lower than those of Dominican female sex workers, but also because they look better and are socially presentable.

I delved into these newspapers with the hope of finding anything related (directly or indirectly) to the aforementioned concepts and terms. Nevertheless, most of my findings were related to cases of gender violence. In response to this, a paralegal official at a human rights NGO for vulnerable groups expressed that Dominicans only pay attention to sex workers' issues when the latter are killed (Rojas 2011; Sosa 2014; Rodriguez-Bloch 2017; *Amnistía Internacional* 2017). Consequently, sex workers are seen as disposable bodies, "outliers and noncitizens" (Kempadoo 2004, 28). His observation also serves as an example of how sexuality functions as ". . . a dense point of exchange of power through which certain bodies emerge as worthy of rights, while others are produced as dangerous contagions that need regulation and discipline" (DasGupta and DasGupta 2018, 6).

This same paralegal also indicated to me that these crimes are often cataloged as *crímenes pasionales* (crimes of passion), falling into two general categories: (1) female CSWs being killed by their romantic partners after the partner realizes the woman is a sex worker, and (2) male CSWs murdering their clients because the client didn't pay the agreed amount of money. The latter type of case included murders of newscaster Claudio Nasco in 2013 (Castillo 2013); director, writer, and producer Micky Bretón in 2009 (*Hoy* 2009); and journalist Víctor Gulias in 2007 (Diaz 2007). Using the term *pasional* to describe an act of violence implies that the person who committed the crime was being irrational and driven by feelings of rage. Yet identifying such crimes as *pasionales* (re)produces a toxic narrative that places men as controlling, abusive, and materialistic. It shows how cases of violence against male CSWs can go under-reported as long as they don't involve a renowned figure.

The described experiences served as the foundation for my research; they shed light on the ways sex work and the people involved in it are addressed on the Island and enabled me to juxtapose the local reality on the ground with the ways that academic literature discusses sex work and related issues. Thereafter, upon returning to the United States, I began to craft my research instruments/questionnaires as well as to plan my next visit to the Island, all informed by this preliminary visit. The aim of this second visit was to conduct formal interviews with NGO staff and with bugarrones themselves. Hence, I prepared a set of thirty-six questions—in addition to a section on demographic data—that sought to capture the subjects' understandings and experiences within the sex work industry.[2]

DE BUGARRONES Y ALGO MÁS . . . (ON *BUGARRONES* AND OTHER MATTERS)

The term "sex worker" or *trabajador/a sexual* became popular in the Dominican Republic around the 1980s with the flourishing of the HIV/AIDS epidemic (Padilla 2007, 15). It sought to identify—or surveil—a great group of people who engaged in sex for money. Nevertheless, and as Padilla indicates, the problem with it is that it tries to homogenize or give a standardized image of sex work that is tied to static social constructs of sex and gender (page 54). Even though the terms "sex worker" and "prostitute" are oftentimes paired together, they should not be treated equally. The first one has an agentic element as it tries to acknowledge the selling of sex as legitimate work, together with the recognition of these people's right to human dignity. It also seeks to communicate that women are not the only ones to offer these services. There are many types of CSWs, in terms of their appearance and catering of services that may change in response to the forces of supply and demand in the global market (Kempadoo 2004, 39; Cabezas 2009, 28).

In the case of Dominican male sex workers, Tabet et al. (1996) drew up a sample of 346 men in order to identify the following general types: (1) the cross dresser, that is, a man who dresses and behaves as a woman; (2) the homosexual, that is, an openly gay man who only has sex with other men; (3) the gigolo, commonly known as the beach boy or a *sanky panky,* that is, a man who sports a tropical fashion (dreadlocks, swimsuits, open Hawaiian shirt or no shirt) and engages in sex with women, and sometimes with men; (4) the bisexual, that is, a man who engages in sex with both women and men; and (5) the heterosexual, that is, a man who only has sex with women. Yet, the population that I am focusing on, the bugarrones, are not explicitly included here, as the word "heterosexual" means having sex with a person from the opposite sex. The term *bugarrón* is a *criollización* of the word "buggery" (Kempadoo 2004, 183), which is mainly tied to the ancient buggery laws that criminalize anal intercourse as an animalistic behavior (Miller 2017). In the words of Rafael Ramírez (1999, 96–98):

> The bugarrón is a man who considers himself to be heterosexual. . . . During sex, he is always the penetrator, both oral and anal. His usage of sexuality is highly ritualized to conserve his manhood and avoid being questioned about it. . . . Invariably, bugarrones are young and have some physical appeal that is valued in *el ambiente*, such as large penises and a manly bearing; they know how to use their sexuality to their advantage.

By performing the penetrator role, the bugarrón then identifies as the *activo* (dominant) partner in sex. The term (or the dominant/submissive system) is intrinsically tied to homosexual culture to indicate who is the "top" and who is the "bottom" person. Although these are sexual positions, they are also positions of power—as one can be physically, economically, or metaphorically "on top" of someone. This type of domination or subordination, for the purposes of this context, dictates what a real man is and how he has to behave in order to be worthy of the title. Australian sociologist, R.W. Connell, labels this as "hegemonic masculinity" (Connell 1995, 77), a type of masculinity that reproduces a heteropatriarchal system (Kempadoo 2004, 1–2). Such structure values and merits men's promiscuity and condemns women's which, in turn, universalizes ". . . relations of power that are intolerant of and oppressive toward sexual desires and practices that are outside or oppose the dominant sexual and gender regimes" (Kempadoo 2004, 9). Smith-Nonini also defines this as body politics; the idealized form of what someone, given a particular context and space, should be (Smith-Nonini 2010, 52–53).

If, by any chance, these men break or contest these values and guidelines, they run the risk of becoming less of a man in front of society. Once a bugarrón is anally penetrated, he becomes a *pasivo*, a term reserved for effeminate and submissive gay men (Thing 2009, 9–10). More colloquially, this man would be called *pájaro* (big bird), *loca* (crazy woman), or *cundango* (faggot) (Reddock 2004, 90–91). While conversing with a family friend about this project, he went on to clearly describe for me what a bugarrón is. He stated, "a real bugarrón hits [from behind]. If he tell you he hits and gets hit too, he lyin'. He a bisexual. And if he only get hit and he like it, it means he a big bird. There's nothin' else to look at." Although the activo/pasivo model seems to reproduce dichotomic heteronormative sexual roles among same-sex partners, scholars have pointed out that there is a third sexual role or identity that allows for fluidity. This is identified in U.S. Latino populations as the *versátil* (versatile) role (Carballo-Diéguez, Dolezal, Nieves, et al. 2004, 159), while in Mexico and Peru these roles are catalogued as *internacionales*—internationals—(Carrier 1977; Carrier 1995; Cantú Jr. 1999; Carballo-Diéguez, Dolezal, Nieves, et al. 2004, 160; Thing 2009, 19; Thing 2010, 817) or *modernos*—modern men—(Cácerez and Rosasco 1999; Carballo-Diéguez, Dolezal, Nieves, et al. 2004, 160), respectively. In simple terms, a versatile man is someone who is confident in receiving and giving anal sex. In the Dominican Republic, the word *versátil* is used by young men on the internet. They market themselves as something "new," "exciting," and "non-conventional." Although a play on words, it is interesting to observe how this third concept is tied with progress, development, and modernity. There is even an element of civilization, because the versátil man is able to adjust to his partners' sexual preferences, even if they are contrary to what the former is used to. Moreover, it can be speculated that the versátil man is un *hombre justo* (fair, just man) with his partner(s) as he is not only receiving pleasure but returning the favor, as well. In this sense, both parties see each other as equals in terms of their sexual needs and capabilities. Equality is the focus of significant discussions among the LGBTQ community where the term *versátil* is employed. Many Dominicans think that gringos are to blame for advocating homosexuality on the Island, including the openly gay U.S. ambassador to the Dominican Republic, Wally Brewster (Londoño 2016; García Marco 2016).

Dominicans have been celebrating and advocating for the recognition of LGBTQ rights on the Island since the sixties (Betances 2013) with the support from local organizations like Colectivo de Gays y Lesbianas Dominicanos (Gay Les Dom), Trans Siempre Amigas (TRANSSA), and the Human Rights

Observatory. This has facilitated multiple public protests (López 2013; *Acento* 2018) and talks with people in power (*Programa de las Naciones Unidas para el Desarrollo, PNUD* 2018) as a way to visibilize the discrimination and violence (physical, mental, and systematic) LGBTQ people suffer in the Dominican Republic (Francisco 2018). Regardless of the aforementioned, the overall Dominican population cannot seem to accept and embrace sexual and gender diversity as part of their national identity. One could argue that this phobia (as well as racism towards Haitians) is one of the legacies—or traumas—of the Trujillo dictatorship (from 1930 to 1961). After all, Trujillo made sure to create and establish a national identity that exalted heteropatriarchy as part of the "true" nation. Hence, homosexuality is seen by most as something foreign and external from what a real Dominican is, and the reason why the U.S. ambassador is such a controversial figure.

Gringos, as well as other foreigners, are the major force in the Dominican pleasure industry—so much so that their presence dictates sex workers' high and low seasons. Their busiest times are the months of July to August, Thanksgiving week, and late December to early January. Throughout these months, sex workers can choose their clients, as well as how much to charge them. Unlike prostitutes, escorts, and other people who exchange sex for money through a more centralized medium (a brothel, a strip club, or a *casa de citas*/hostess bar) that dictates their fares and takes a percentage of their earnings, sex workers do so in a more independent fashion. They actively look for their clients (at bars, on the streets, in restaurants, coffee shops, etc.) and establish their own rates according to the services requested by the client and the bugarrón's own sense of value in the market. When low season arrives, and the number of foreigners decreases substantially, these male CSWs must conform with what the client can offer them at the time. One of the main reasons why CSWs prefer an international clientele is because the value of foreign currency is likely to be higher than the Dominican peso. Hence, even if they give substantial discounts to clients during the low season, sex workers could still be able to earn a decent living.

In 2016, the tourism industry was responsible for 17 percent of the national gross domestic product (GDP) (*Diario Turístico de la República Dominicana* 2017) in the Dominican Republic, positioning the Island "as the ninth largest economy in Latin America . . . and a GDP world ranking of 74" (Caplan, Little, and Garces-King 2016, 193). A quick look at the two tables published by the Dominican Office of National Statistics show how the tourism sector in the Island has grown since 2011.

Both table 2.1 and table 2.2 use hotels and other tourist-related establishments as their units of measure. They also include an estimate on "indirect" jobs that have also benefitted by such growth, like taxi drivers, restaurant and

Table 2.1. DOMINICAN REPUBLIC: Evolution of the Tourism Sector by Year, According to Main Indicators, 2011–2015[1]

Main indicators	*2011*	*2012*	*2013*	*2014*	*2015*
Hotel occupancy rates (%)	69.3	70.3	71.7	74.8	75.5
Hotel rooms	66,790	66,323	68,542	68,840	69,816
Tourism income (US millions)	4,352.8	4,736.3	5,125	5,637	6,153
Total generated jobs by the tourism activity	201,597	201,235	216,543	247,025	254,146
Direct jobs generated by the tourism activity	57,599	57,496	61,869	70,578	71,686
Indirect jobs generated by the tourism activity	143,998	143,739	154,674	176,447	182,460

[1]This is a short version of the table. For a complete table, please check the 2016 National Statistic Report at the official site of the Dominican National Statistics Office (ONE) on http://www.one.gob.do/Categoria/Publicaciones/1973#

Table 2.2. DOMINICAN REPUBLIC: Number of Establishments (E) and Tourist Accommodation Rooms (R) Per Year, According to Province (P) and Municipality (M), 2011–2015[1]

	2011	*2011*	*2012*	*2012*	*2013*	*2013*	*2014*	*2014*	*2015*	*2015*
Province and municipality	E	R	E	R	E	R	E	R	E	R
Total	724	67,289	789	66,019	791	64,397	724	69,596	724	70,060
National District (P)	128	6,441	153	7,110	153	7,110	147	7,440	148	7,255
Boca Chica (M)	51	1,916	52	1,928	52	1,928	50	1,928	50	1,928
La Romana (P)	14	820	16	881	16	881	13	1,123	13	1,125
La Altagracia (P)	88	33,589	102	35,019	102	33,387	102	37,420	100	38,066
Bayahíbe (M)	8	2,949	9	2,966	9	2,966	9	2,966	10	3,210
Punta Cana (M)	4	1,180	8	1,638	7	1,153	12	2,796	10	2,620
Puerto Plata (P)	173	14,275	181	11,666	181	11,986	145	12,401	145	12,541
Puerto Plata (M)	9	177	9	177	9	177	9	177	10	367
Sosúa (M)	72	4,204	75	3,564	75	3,864	61	3,763	59	3,663

[1]This is a short version of the table. For a complete table, please check the 2016 National Statistic Report at the official site of the Dominican National Statistics Office (ONE) on http://www.one.gob.do/Categoria/Publicaciones/1973#

nightclub owners, and so on. Here, the word "indirect" means that these jobs are affected, to a certain degree, by the flow of tourists. Although sex workers are also affected by the same dynamic, they are not included here as they are part of the informal sector. Their labor is considered "informal" because it is not taxable or controlled by the state.

As a result of social stigma, systemic oppression, and constant surveillance, sex workers in tourist areas have adopted different strategies in order to fight back and earn their money. One such strategy is that instead of establishing a purely monetary relationship with their clients, they resort to more romantic approaches (like taking them to restaurants, discos, and a plethora of other places) as a way to secure their client and have them visit the Island more often, send remittances from abroad—as the Dominican peso's economic value is less than that of the Euro and/or the U.S. dollar—or even ask for their visa so that the CSWs can join the foreigner abroad. Although the person who ends up paying for everything is the client, a bond is made. Researchers have suggested that, in this case, we cannot refer to this as "*sex* tourism" but as "*romance* tourism" because it involves feelings and emotions (Cabezas 2004, 991).

Sex work thus requires both physical and emotional labor (Hochschild 1983, ix, 7; Kang 2010, 22)—the first, one because it is the type of job that is carried out with the use of their bodies, and the second, because it involves a deeper connection with the client. Since bugarrones are aware of this, they are what Dominicans call *unos tígueres*—tigers, street smart—(Reddock 2004, 90–91; Horn 2014, 41). They see their chance and they take it. By thinking of their clients as effeminate, they use the same tactics they use to conquer any woman: *dándole cotorra y muela* (sweet-talking them). Once they have a secure client that will meet with them numerous times, they start pulling out the heavy guns: *los cuentos*, or random little stories or white lies (Padilla 2007, 39) about how they got robbed on the way and cannot pay their bus fare to go back home; that they are thinking of applying to college but the books are too expensive; that one of their relatives is sick and they need money for medicines, and so on. The use of these tactics assures them of extra cash, and it communicates to the foreigner that they are struggling, vulnerable humans—not only an erect, walking penis. If seen from a political-economy lens, it is now the colonized exploiting the colonizer, the savage dominating the developed, by turning the neo-liberal system against its creators. As Julia Suárez-Krabbe puts it, they have mastered the master's tools (Suárez-Krabbe 2015, 17).

¿UN TRABAJO FÁCIL? (AN EASY JOB?)

Although I made several attempts to recruit a significant and representative sample of bugarrones on my own (i.e., by sharing information about the project on different web-based platforms used to offer these types of services), my outreach resulted in a few exchanges with potential research subjects, but no concrete interviews. Nevertheless, this exercise enabled me to make several significant observations about my population. One was that the internet gave these men a sense of safety: to communicate with me online did not involve communicating in public locations that are surveilled by police officers. In addition to that, online communication allowed them to protect (or hide) their identity and create a new one by using a nickname or username allegorical to either their sexual organs/physical attributes, or their sexual preferences or role(s). Furthermore, the internet provided these men with a cheap method for reaching their clientele, as they did not have to invest much materially in order to meet clients.

In this case, I use the term "invest" to express both the tangible and intangible side of the exchange with the potential client. For example, by using the internet these men save money by not having to go from one place to another looking for clients, or by not having to buy their drinks at a bar while waiting for a potential client. Additionally, they don't have to put much effort into their appearances (i.e., the clothes that they are wearing, their cologne, hair, etc.) because they can send a picture that was previously taken. Therefore, the internet provides them with a cost-effective way to attract clients. Moreover, it also allows these men to talk with a larger pool of potential clients by forwarding the same message to different people. Internet communications also help formalize norms of accountability and responsibility between the parties involved because things like fares for services are written down.

On one of the first Friday afternoons of the year, I met with a man whom I identify as John Salchichón (a retired bugarrón) at the entrance of La Zona Colonial. From there, he took me to a safe space where I would be able to conduct my interviews with a group of MSM sex workers for whom John acted as a health promoter and facilitator. The place was not that far from the main street (El Conde), yet it looked very different: the streets had trash, the outside walls of the houses looked dirty, music came from all over—from houses, *colmadones*,[3] passersby, and so on. There were children playing barefoot on the street, and dogs and roosters walking alongside people. Most of the people that I saw in this area had visible Afro-Caribbean characteristics (i.e., they were dark-skinned with braided or kinky long hair, simulating the image of the *sanky panky* or the beach boy), in addition to sporting a similar fashion style. Men wore loose jeans, brand-name or extremely clean sneakers, and polo shirts. Most of them were gathered at the *colmadón* as a group or around their motorcycles (*motos* or *pasolas*). The women I saw in this area were wearing either tight-fitting clothes or very short, revealing outfits that showcased their voluptuous frames. In addition to that, most of them had their hair in a *tubi* (a doobie wrap), which meant that it had recently been done at the hair salon and they were saving it to unwrap later that night.

Once there, John introduced me to a group of five men who showed interest in the project. He also joined the interview process, and thus, my final sample size consisted of six men. I interviewed each man separately, and the procedure took around thirty minutes to one hour per participant, depending on how thorough and detailed their answers were. In order to protect their privacy, I never asked for their names.[4] Nevertheless, I did ask for their pseudonyms to see how they were/are known in the business and altered them to decrease the chances of them being identified by any reader. Such men are identified in table 2.3 (which follows) as John Salchichón (currently retired from sex work but willing to participate),[5] The Giant, and Lil' Cheeks. These men's pseudonyms represent their physical characteristics and their role as MSM practitioners. They also depict, to a certain degree, how masculine they are to the public—as the latter are the ones who name them.

The men of my sample share demographic similarities with those included in a report made in 2012 by Giancarlo Martínez Blandino and Francisca Ferreira, which aimed to educate the MSM population on HIV/AIDS prevention and treatment. With this in mind, one can assume that these bugarrones are a small but significant representation of the overall Dominican MSM sex-work universe. In addition to these similarities with the literature, the narrative of using sex work as a tactic to satisfy their immediate economic needs (Cabezas 2009: 120) was recurrent in almost all the participants' testimonies. For example, Dewars (a dark-skinned, thirty-seven-year-old heterosexual man with four children and fourteen years in the field as an activo) shared that, before engaging in sex with other men, he saw this activity as an effortless way to earn money. However, once he saw himself alone with another man, he realized that it wasn't such an easy job. To him, it was *un trago amargo* (a bitter pill). Similarly, The Giant (a light-skinned, forty-year-old, bisexual man with ten years of experience as an activo) explained to me that, even though he has worked in multiple sectors and industries, sex work is the only substantial source of income with which he can provide for his family.

Another participant, Diorys (an *indio,* twenty-four-year-old heterosexual Christian man with seven years of experience as an activo), saw his earnings as *dinero diabólico* (diabolical money) because you can earn a lot in a second and have nothing in the next. Other participants echoed Diorys's opinion, admitting that sex work permits you to earn money fast—because you receive the money directly from the client after the service is done—but not in an easy way, as they are doing something they do not enjoy. Hence, it is the ability of making money at a fast rate that makes this profession popular among low-income groups or those with immediate economic needs. As a result, many of

Table 2.3. Samples' Sociodemographic Characteristics

	#1	*#2*	*#3*	*#4*	*#5*	*#6*
Pseudonym	N/A	N/A	N/A	The Giant	Lil' Cheeks	John Salchichón
Age	29	24	37	40	33	45
Level of education	Eighth grade	Seventh grade	Fourth grade	Ninth grade	Sixth grade	High school
Sexual orientation	Hetero	Hetero	Hetero	Bisexual	Hetero	Bisexual
Marital status	Single	In a relationship	In partnership	Single	Divorced	Free union
No. of children	1	0	4	2	1	5
Religion	N/A	Christian	N/A	N/A	Catholic	Catholic
Years of experience	14 years	7 years	14 years	10 years	20+ years	30 years
MSM identity/role	Activo	Activo	Activo	Activo	Pasivo	Activo

Other job experience	Cook	N/A	Mechanic, construction	Barbershop, brewery, hotelier sector, security guard, Free-Trade Zone	Bartender	Bartender, table dancer, stripper
Reason for being MSM	Needed money	Needed money	Needed money	Needed money	Needed money	Needed money
Socioeconomic status	Poor	Normal	Poor	Middle class	Middle class	Middle class
Race	Black	Indio	Black	White	White	White
Skin color	Dark	Tanned	Dark	Light	Light	Light
Work place	Gay bars at the Zona Colonial	Bars and discos at the Zona Colonial	El Conde	Gay bar	El Conde	Retired

Source: Generated by Author

these bugarrones engage in substance abuse (drugs, alcohol) when on duty. Brayan (a dark-skinned, twenty-nine-year-old heterosexual man with fourteen years of experience as an a*ctivo,* and a child of his own) said that, although he does not use drugs or alcohol, he uses sexual potency pills because:

> The gay man always has the mentality that you have to. . . . You have to do your work for them and hit them hard. . . . They want for me to suck them and I don't do that. They want for me to make out with them and I can't . . . I tell them that I don't like [those things]. They want to penetrate me and I don't like that either. . . . That's why it's better for me to stay poor. If I don' like one thing, I prefer not to do it.

Brayan's statement sheds light on numerous topics (i.e., hypermasculinity, the concept of a "real" bugarrón, and the balancing of one's economic needs over one's values) delineated in previous sections. Nonetheless, the following segment of the chapter connects his (and other men's) statement(s) with the three elements of my title—(in)visibility, masculinities, and same-sex performances—that are palpable and overarching throughout these men's narratives. Of course, these are not the only recurrent topics in their responses. Yet, given the purposes and limitations of this chapter, they are the only ones I can directly examine.

(IN)VISIBILITY

As noted previously, I use the term "invisibilization" to highlight the unique process of exclusion MSM sex workers face in the Dominican Republic. Such process happens in an implicit way, mostly by the persistence of crímenes pasionales as the only cases where sex workers are included in the local media. Consequently, questions regarding the ways media outlets present sex work(ers) were asked of the participants.

To these, many sex workers expressed that if local media were to showcase the reality of sex work and its participants, it would improve the public's perception of it, as it would make their struggles and reasons for becoming sex workers apparent. They added that more media coverage, done the right way, could also gain them empathy from the public, as most Dominicans are economically struggling. Furthermore, it would educate Islanders on issues like human rights, community issues, police brutality, and equality. In other words, bugarrones saw news outlets as sources of empowerment for populations at risk, like them. Not even once did these men mention the State or the government as responsible for this. One reason for this might be because of how corrupt Dominican government has shown itself to be, in addition to the treatment these men—and other sex workers—get from police officers while doing their job.

In addition to that, the men in my sample indicated that they were affiliated with an institution John Salchichón works for as a health promoter. The organization provides them with condoms, free HIV/AIDS tests, and other prevention techniques so that they can take care of their bodies while offering sexual services. After all, sex workers see their bodies as commodities in a system where they are always—because of their lack of resources—at a disadvantage. Despite the institutions' efforts to protect these men, more could (and should) be done. Instead of only targeting MSM sex workers' physical bodies, institutions could offer them a space where they can meet with other male sex workers to share their experiences and foster community within and between them. As a result, a sense of belonging could emerge and possibly present them with the consolidation of a male sex workers' union, much like female sex workers have institutionalized (*Global Network of Sex Work Projects*).

On the other hand, when directly asked if they felt invisible in the Dominican society, most of these men (except for one) indicated that they feel "normal." Normal in the sense that they are able to approach potential clients and discuss fares face-to-face with them. In Diorys's words, he says that he feels:

> Normal. Err'one respect me and like me and all because, in reality, although I do what I do, I am a regular *tíguere* [tiger]. I mean, not that I am a tíguere [that robs or does bad things] but I try to be with err'one: tigueres, *parigüayos* [creolization of "party watcher," a ninny] . . . Err'one.

Here, Diorys emphasizes that he is a good kind of tíguere and that, because of this, people respect him even as his bugarrón background has gone public. However, Diorys's case is a rare one, as most of the men of my sample indicated that they keep their sex-worker background a secret from their family and friends. They feel that, because of all the stigma around sex work, they will be cast out of their inner circles. This is why these men feel safe offering their services in enclosed spaces (i.e., gay bars/discos or the internet) as there is less probability that they encounter a close friend/relative in there.

Race proved to be an element of hypervisibility, especially for the two dark-skinned men in my sample, Brayan and Dewars. Whenever their neighbors saw them with white male foreigners, the CSWs would receive comments tied to the color of their skin and the assumption of their hypersexuality. Dewars expressed feeling publicly bullied by his neighbors, which made him overtly conscious about the types of clients he associates with. In order to minimize suspicions and the kinds of comments he might receive from others, he tries to pair up with foreigners that don't look too gay or effeminate. His target is the type of man who looks "normal" or that can pass as a regular friend in the eyes of others. Yet, other elements (such as a large age gap) between the client and the sex worker also play a big role, which, together with race, makes these men overtly visible to locals. Consequently, bugarrones run the risk of damaging their "manly" reputation, their family,[6] or other things they deemed valuable by the simple act of being seen with men too different from them.

MASCULINITIES

Five out of the six men in my sample identified as activos. They also referred to themselves as "normal," "100 percent man," and heterosexual, because they only offered penetrative services to their clients. However, some of them admitted to offering "extra services" so long as the client did not look like a total *loca,* too effeminate, or with too many obvious mannerisms. Some of these included guided tours around the historical center, holding hands, and/or kissing. These are primarily requested by the client, and not offered firsthand by sex workers. Yet, the latter are always up for negotiating, as they can also charge more for those services. During our interview, The Giant explained how he manages to consent on what services he gets to provide his clients with, and under what conditions. He said:

> Sometimes [I would] give them a tour, they ask for it themselves. Sometimes they only want sex, and other times they want to stay with you. The client speaks for himself. I always do [what the client asks]. What I don't like is that, if they tell you how much they're going to pay you, and then they decide to pay you less. Or those who [tell you that they] want one thing and then tell you that "no, I'd better penetrate you" something that's out [of the deal]. . . . Understand? Always talk'd. [When that happens, I get] upset because sometimes those [clients] don't deviate from what they are used to do in the way they are used to do it. And that's it, we get to an agreement that things are done this way and that's it.

For the male sex workers in my sample, consent seems to be a natural thing between them and their clients. Bugarrones's choices seem to be respected by their clients. Nevertheless, there are some customers that do their best to tempt the sex workers and make them break their rigid rules. Instances where the client offers them enormous amounts of money or tries to get them drunk or drugged were common in my sample. Yet, the five activo men stated they have never allowed another man to penetrate them. They portrayed themselves to me as being confident about turning down any propositions that went against their persona and definition of a Dominican man. Thus, although these men acknowledged that they were living in precarious situations, they were able to act according to their own moral values and beliefs. In a way, the fact that these men could negotiate and consent with their clients indicates that they are not powerless.

Although those that I interviewed did not want their clients to penetrate them, kissing and holding hands are another story. Some bugarrones might engage in these types of affectionate gestures with their clients only if they are in private spaces (i.e., the bedroom), dark spaces (i.e., a bar or a disco), and/or spaces in which they usually don't have access to by themselves because of their socioeconomic status (i.e., a fancy restaurant). All of these serve as "safe spaces" for MSM sex workers as they assume that no one who knows them will be there. Therefore, bugarrones are able to both keep their clients happy and protect their manly reputations. To this, Diorys comments:

> I ain't, ain't gonna offer a part of my body that I know that later on won't make me feel like a man. Yet, maybe a lot of people will say "No, but this guy considers himself a man? Because he fucks gay men. . . ." And dis'n dat. But I do feel like a man because, until today, thank God, I haven't given my ass [to other men], understand? And sorry for the word, but I haven't sucked a penis nor will I ever do it. And I think that the day I do that, God have mercy on me, God [should] punish me, really.

If one takes Connell's concept of hegemonic masculinity and applies it to the men in my sample, one can see that they are trying to embody that, but they are not quite there yet. They still have a lot to lose, whether they decide to let everyone in their circle know about the nature of their jobs or if they decide to leave sex work. Henceforth, these men are what the author identifies as "complicit." Complicit in the sense that these men participate in a heteropatriarchal system, but they are not able to change the rules to their advantage. Nevertheless, by differentiating themselves from effeminate men (by shaming them) they are able to position themselves as the second-best masculine man. An example of this is these men's attachment to the activo/pasivo model—as a way to position themselves above their clients—in terms of sexuality and desirability.

On a deeper level, however, there is a social, physical, visible element attached to it that has been addressed by these sex workers. To them (as well as to other people) activos are always seen as masculine or the man in the relationship, while pasivos are thought of as the effeminate part or the woman in the partnership, regardless of the sexual role they perform privately. The abovementioned, in my opinion, presents an interesting breaking point in these men's narratives. By rejecting effeminate-looking men as clients, one can assume that bugarrones either lower their masculine/macho-man behaviors as a mechanism to attract the "right" kind of customers or that they decide to engage with effeminate clients anyway. This represents an ongoing balance of power for MSM sex workers, as they are constantly looking to protect their reputations but also earn a living.

SAME-SEX PERFORMANCES

The word "performance" does not have a direct translation in Spanish. Therefore, I used both the terms *actuación* (act) and *representación* (representation) when asking the participants about how they saw their sexual role and/or identity when they were with other men. Additionally, I asked them about for whom and how they carried it out. With the exception of two participants, the men in my sample agreed that they, indeed, engaged in performing an identity that could go on for as long as they kept in contact with their customers. Dewars explained that "*e' como tene' una novia*" (it's like having a girlfriend) as they have to call their clients to see how they are doing and engage in a conversation that does not always revolve around asking their clients for money. Ergo, in this phase, they mostly do emotional labor.

Together with this kind of labor comes what they call *romance* tourism as there is something more than sex that keeps the foreigner going back to this Caribbean paradise. Surprisingly, the term *romance tourism* is usually cited in the literature as something that emerges from heterosexual exchanges between sex workers and their clients. The concept reproduces a heteronormative system between the parties involved, indicating that the less powerful party (the sex worker) is the one who initiates the romantic gestures towards the other individual, and thus, could be seen as "the woman" in the relationship. My goal was to understand the way these men felt towards their regular or long-term clients. When I asked them directly if they have ever developed feelings towards their clients, the participants stated that they did not. However, when asked differently ("Have you ever felt [emotion/sentiment/feeling] towards any of your clients?") I was able to capture more complex answers. Four of these men indicated that they've felt a lot of respect and gratitude towards some of their clients, as the latter have been able to give them a hand in difficult times. Brayan even said that he is friends with one of his clients and that they keep in touch regularly, as platonic friends.

The remaining two bugarrones of my sample stated that they have come to really like and love some of their clients. In the case of Dewars, he explained that it has only happened once to him, with a Boricua[7] man with whom he had a relationship for thirteen years. The other man who acknowledged developing this kind of sentiment for one of his clients was John Salchichón, who also had a relationship with a Boricua man. Attachment, then, becomes unavoidable when there is a constant exchange of affection—be it sexual and/or romantic—between these men. Thus, I wondered if these men's denial of developing any kind of feelings towards their clients emerged as a defense mechanism to maintain and restate their dominion over "the other." After all, as the popular refrain goes, the one who loves the most in a relationship is thought to be the less powerful one, as they can be easily manipulated by the other party.

Subsequently, and although both Dewars and John Salchichón shared developing romantic feelings for their clients, they also emphasized the fact that they continued to perform the activo role in the relationship, always. Thus, by holding on to the activo role, they were still stating their manhood—and power—to others and to themselves. Moreover, this adds another level of complexity when we talk about same-sex performances, in the sense that these performances might not even be executed for the pleasure of others (the clients) but for the bugarrones' sake, to maintain the little control they have over their bodies and lives.

Moreover, and taking into consideration my own positionality (Skelton 2001, 89; Clifford, French and Valentine 2010, 166; Yakushko, Badjee, Mallory and Wang 2011): a white, well-educated, cisgender, young Dominican woman; and the market value I represented to these men: a U.S. citizenship that translates to international mobility and access to dollars; their words could be read in many other valid ways. For example, one could argue that the reason why these men held on so strongly to heteronormative definitions of gender and sexuality was because they wanted me to perceive them and present them as real men through my work, regardless of their occupation. Thus, in addition to performing for their clients, they could have been putting up a performance for me as well, or for the person they saw me as at the moment of our exchanges. For them, I was not only a researcher but a *female* researcher. As a response to this, as I interviewed them, the bugarrones acted courteously towards me, making sure that the chair I sat in was comfortable or that my (straightened) hair[8] didn't get wet from the rain. By being seen in public with me, these men increased their value in the eyes of locals and passersby. Our interaction, in a sense, could be seen as a game of objectifying the Other for power or, in my case, for knowledge.

The abovementioned observations show the ways MSM sex workers perform the different definitions and expectations of Dominican masculinity to restate that, no matter their sexual practices, they are still "normal" men. With their words and actions, they showed that their precarious situation does not limit them when it comes to saying no to whatever they perceived as unnatural or abnormal. Still, other elements like pride, self-consciousness, and a binary interpretation of gender relations are also part of these MSM sex workers' responses to the questions I asked them. Without any of these elements, one could assume that the men in my sample could adopt a versátil or a pasivo role with their customers more easily. This adaptability shows that their economic precarity is necessary but not sufficient to make these men offer their bodies to foreigners. And that other factors motivate or influence the manner in which they offer sex work.

CONCLUSIONS

The present work explored the ways and reasons MSM commercial sex workers or bugarrones are made invisible in the Dominican society by primarily focusing on semi-structured interviews held with them. This was done as a way to show other approaches—aside from a public health approach—that can be adopted to study and understand at-risk populations. By focusing on these men's experiences, I sought to give light to a more humane side of sex work(ers). Additionally, the present study sheds light on some of the disconnections between academic, institutional, and local media discourses around the topic. Local news outlets, as well as Dominican pop-culture products, are a great way to explore the present status of this society. They represent what people consume on a day-to-day basis, either by choice or by imposition. Henceforth, by using social and feminist studies' theories to analyze these mediums, we develop a critical understanding of what is taking place on the Island. The latter could lead to a collective social empowerment with the potential to transform the ways in which information is (re)produced in the Dominican Republic. Subsequently, it would allow for the inclusion of marginalized Others into the national narrative, resulting in the plurality, or multiplicity, of Foucault's "good citizen."

Because of its reduced scope and sample size, this study should be seen as a jumping-off point to other researchers interested in the topic of sex work(ers) in the Caribbean and other regions. Topics such as the balance of power, the processes and/or choice of (in)visibilization as a survival technique, the bending of the activo/pasivo model in terms of the Dominican Republic, and the client-sex worker platonic/long-term relationships require further in-depth study. Some of the future directions that could be taken include the study of college students who resort to selling their bodies to pay for tuition, the supportive networks between MSM sex workers and their female partners, dating apps for the promotion of sexual services, and how Venezuelan migration to the Dominican Republic is affecting the demand for Dominican sex workers.

As expressed previously by the men in my sample, sex work is a complicated and complex topic as it goes beyond economic parameters. Moreover, being a CSW requires more than just a healthy, desirable, consumable body. Hence, by allowing ourselves to understand the factors and reasons why people rely on this activity as their primary source of income (while being aware of its many risks), it allows us to evaluate the ways we can think of alternatives to help vulnerable groups. By doing this, we will stop invisibilizing the people and the problems around them. Subsequently, this could lead to a more holistic, representative, and significant drafting of public policies, research studies, and community initiatives that are much needed in the Dominican Republic.

NOTES

1. "Real" Dominican men are thought to be serious men who provide for their families. In addition to that, it is assumed that they have multiple female partners—aside from their wives or "official" partners; assumed because it is suspected but never—at least not most of the time—corroborated. This can be tied to the figure of Rafael L. Trujillo, a Dominican dictator who was known for spending many a young girl's first night of marriage with her, if he found her attractive and/or sexually appealing.

2. Protocol #H17-302, approved on December 27, 2017. Valid until December 21, 2018.

3. It is the revamped version of a *colmado* or *bodega* in the sense that it sells alcohol, in addition to grocery goods. Furthermore, it also provides the client with chairs and tables where they can sit with their friends and enjoy *una fría* or "a cold one," meaning a beer.

4. Although the consent form asks for their name and their signature, it was not a requisite for them to sign the consent form. This was done as a way to protect their identities, confidentiality, and privacy, in accordance with IRB protocols and guidelines.

5. Since at the time of the interview he expressed being retired but willing to participate, the answers that he provided me with were based on when he used to engage in the profession.

6. These men's parents were not aware of the men's involvement in sex work as *bugarrones*. Rather, the men disguised themselves as tour guides, security guards at bars, and so on. Even though they indicated to me that they did not care if they were to find out, they still refused or omitted to tell them, out of respect for them. However, some of these men's romantic partners were aware of their work environment.

7. Another term for Puerto Rican.

8. In the Dominican Republic, hair texture is a sign of racial superiority. Usually, people with curly hair are associated with Haiti and Africa, and are thought of as black and dumb, and therefore curly hair is regarded as a bad thing to be born with. Straight hair, on the contrary, is associated with white Europeans, who are seen as progressive and smart. Hence, straight hair is desired for its social interpretation of intelligence and development. For more on this topic, please see Ginette Candelarios's "Black Behind the Ears" (2007), which focuses on blackness in the Dominican Republic.

WORKS CITED

Bastidas, Felipe and Marbella Torrealba. "Definición y desarrollo del concepto "proceso de invisibilización" para el análisis social. Una aplicación preliminar a algunos casos de la sociedad venezolana." *Espacio Abierto* 23, no. 3, (2014): 515–533.

Betanes, Diuris. "El orgullo gay en la República Dominicana." *Observatorio Político Dominicano, OPD* (Santo Domingo, DR), Aug. 5, 2013.

Brennan, Denise. "Women Work, Men Sponge, and Everyone Gossips: Macho Men and Stigmatized/ing Women in a Sex Tourist Town." *Anthropological Quarterly* 77, no. 4, (2004): 705–733.

Cabezas, Amalia L. "Between Love and Money: Sex, Tourism, and Citizenship in Cuba and the Dominican Republic." *Signs* 29, no. 4 (2004): 987–1015.

Cabezas, Amalia L. *Economies of Desire: Sex and Tourism in Cuba and the Dominican Republic*. Philadelphia: Temple University Press, 2009.

Cáceres, C. F. and A. M. Rosasco. "The Margin has Many Sides: Diversity Among Gay and Homosexually Active Men in Lima." *Culture, Health, and Sexuality* 1, no. 3 (1999): 261–275.

Candelario, Ginetta E. B. *Black behind the Ears: Dominican Racial Identity from Museums to Beauty Shops.* Durham, NC: Duke University Press, 2007.

Cantú, Lionel Jr. "Border Crossings: Mexican Men and the Sexuality of Migration." PhD dissertation, University of California-Irvine, 1999.

Caplan, Susan, Tariana V. Little, and Jasmine Garces-King. "Stigma About Mental Illness Among Multidisciplinary Health Care Providers in the Dominican Republic," *International Perspectives in Psychology: Research, Practice, Consultation* 5, no. 3 (2016): 192–206.

Carballo-Diéguez, Alex, Curtis Dolezal, Luis Nieves, et al. "Looking for a Tall, Dark, Macho Man . . . Sexual-role Behaviour Variations in Latino Gay and Bisexual Men." *Culture, Health & Sexuality* 6, no. 2 (2004): 159–171.

Carrier, J. M. "Sex-role Preferences as an Explanatory Variable in Homosexual Behaviour." *Archives of Sexual Behaviour* 6, (1977): 53–65.

Carrier, J. *De Los Otros: Intimacy and Homosexuality Among Mexican Men.* New York: Columbia University Press, 1995.

Castillo, Altagracia. "Asesino de Claudio Nasco dice este nunca le pagaba completo (lea aquí el expediente)." *El Día* (Santo Domingo, DR), Dec. 18, 2013.

Clifford, Nicholas, Shaun French, and Gill Valentine. *Key Methods in Geography.* London: SAGE Publications Ltd, 2010.

Cohen, J. "HIV/AIDS: Latin America & Caribbean. Dominican Republic: The Sun. The Sand. The Sex." *Science* 313, no. 5786, (2006): 474.

Compres, Tiffany. "Labor of Love: Using International Labor Law to Achieve Human Rights for Women Sex Workers in the Dominican Republic." *Georgetown Journal of International Law* 40, no. 3 (2009): 1027–1042.

"Comunidad LGBTI dominicana reclama respeto e inclusi6n." *Acento* (Santo Domingo, DR), July 8, 2018.

Connell, R. W. *Masculinities*. Los Angeles: University of California Press, 1995.

DasGupta, Rohit K. and Debanuj DasGupta, *Queering Digital India.* Edinburg: Edinburg University Press, 2018.

De Moya, Antonio E. "Power Games and Totalitarian Masculinity in the Dominican Republic." In *Interrogating Caribbean Masculinities: Theoretical and Empirical Analyses*, edited by Rhoda Reddock, 68–102. Kingston, Jamaica: University of the West Indies Press, 2004.

Fieser, Ezra. "Un Paraíso para la prostitución en República Dominicana." *El Nuevo Herald* (Miami, FL), Feb. 2, 2013.

Francisco, Juan Alberto. "La comunidad LGBT se desangra en República Dominicana." *Observatorio de Derechos Humanos para Grupos Vulnerabilizados, ODHGV* (Santo Domingo, DR), Aug. 1, 2018.

García Marco, Daniel. "Cómo el embajador gay de EE.UU. ayuda a compatir la homofobia en República Dominicana (y enfada a la Iglesia)." *BBC Mundo* (London, UK), April 9, 2016.

Horn, Maja. *Masculinity after Trujillo: The Politics of Gender in the Dominican Republic.* Gainsville: University Press of Florida, 2014.

International Justice Mission. "Commercial Sexual Exploitation of Children in the Dominican Republic." Official report. Washington, DC, 2015.

Jiménez, Juan Carlos. "Trabajadoras sexuales dominicanas se quejan que venezolanas las desplazan con tarifa más baja." *El Caribe* (Santo Domingo, DR), Jan. 27, 2017.

Kang, Miliann. *The Managed Hand.* Berkeley: University of California Press, 2010.

Kempadoo, Kamala. *Sexing the Caribbean: Gender, Race, and Sexual Labor.* New York: Routledge, 2004.

Londoño, Ernesto. "Gay Pride and Prejudice in Dominican Republic." *New York Times* (New York, NY), April 4, 2016.

Lopez, Ezequiel Abiu. "Desfile gay dominicano exige erradicar agresiones," Associated Press (New York, NY), June 30, 2013.

Martínez Blandino, Giancarlo and Francisca Ferreira. "Proyecto Hombre Seguro: Reporte Final de Investigación." Institutional report, Santo Domingo, DR, 2012.

Miller, Al. "The plain truth about the buggery law," *Jamaica Observer* (Kingston, JA), July 31, 2017.

"MODEMU Founded." *Global Network of Sex Work Projects: Promoting Health and Human Rights.* Last modified November 1, 2015. http://www.nswp.org/timeline/event/modemu-founded

"Organizaciones LGBTI exponen situación derechos humanos a legisladora dominicana." *Programa de las Naciones Unidas para el Desarrollo, PNUD* (Santo Domingo, DR), April 17, 2018.

Padilla, Mark. *Caribbean Pleasure Industry: Tourism, Sexuality, and AIDS in the Dominican Republic.* Chicago: University of Chicago Press, 2007.

Padilla, Mark, Daniel Castellanos, Vincent Guilamo-Ramos, et al. "Stigma, social inequality, and HIV risk disclosure among Dominican male sex workers." *Social Science & Medicine* 67, no. 3, (2008): 380–388.

Pardais, Leah. "Human Rights Situation of Female Sex Workers in the Americas." *Human Rights Brief,* March 24, 2017. http://hrbrief.org/2017/03/human-rights-situation-female-sex-workers-americas/

Pope, Z., D. Hodge, Y. Donastorg, et al. "Sexual risk behaviors and prevalence of sexually transmitted diseases in a cohort of Dominican men who have sex with men." *International Journal of Infectious Diseases*, 21, (2014): 424–424.

Ramírez, Rafael. *What it means to be a man: Reflections on Puerto Rican Masculinity.* New Brunswick: Rutgers University Press, 1999.

"Rapero admire asesinó a Micky Bretón por violar acuerdo sexual." *Hoy* (Santo Domingo, DR), Nov. 3, 2009.

"República Dominica: Terrible asesinato de mujer transgénero, es necesaria la protección frente a la discriminación." *Amnistía Internacional.* Last modified June 6, 2017. https://www.es.amnesty.org/en-que-estamos/noticias/noticia/articulo/republica-dominicana-terrible-asesinato-de-mujer-transgenero-es-necesaria-la-proteccion-frente/

Rojas, Lissette. "Asesinatos brutales de trabajadoras sexuales dominicanas," *Acento* (Santo Domingo, DR), April 6, 2011.

Russell Hochschild, Arlie. *The Managed Heart.* Berkeley: University of California Press, 1983.

Sanchez Taylor, Jacqueline. "Female Sex Tourism: A Contradiction in Terms?" *Feminist Review*, 83, (2006): 42–59.

Santiago Díaz, Adonis. "Matan de 32 puñaladas al periodista Víctor Gulias." *Diario Libre* (Santo Domingo, DR), March 29, 2007.

Skelton, Tracey. "Cross-Cultural Research: Issues of Power, Positionality and 'Race.'" In *Qualitative Methodologies for Geographers,* edited by Melanie Limb and Claire Dwyer. London: Arnold, 2001.

Smith-Nonini, Sandy. "Repression's Repercussions: Pragmatic Solidarity and the Body Politic." In *Healing the Body Politic: El Salvador's Popular Struggle for Health Rights from Civil war to Neoliberal Peace*. New Brunswick: Rutgers University Press, 2010.

Sosa, José Rafael. "Muere homosexual atacaron en hotel." *El Nacional*. (Santo Domingo, DR), Nov. 1, 2014.

Suárez-Krabbe, Julia. *Race, Rights, and Rebels: Alternatives to Human Rights and Development from the Global South.* London: Rowman & Littlefield International Ltd., 2015.

Tabet, Stephen R., E. Antonio de Moya, King Rosado Holmes, et al. "Sexual Behaviors and Risk Factors for HIV Infection among Men Who Have Sex with Men in the Dominican Republic." *AIDS* 10, no. 2 (1996): 201–206.

Thing, James. "Entre Maricones, Machos y Gays: Globalization and the Construction of Sexual Identities Among Queer Mexicanos." PhD dissertation, University of Southern California, 2009.

Thing, James. "Gay, Mexican and Immigrant: Intersecting Identities Among Gay Men in Los Angeles." *Social Identities* 16, no. 6 (2010): 809–831.

"Turismo aportó el 17 percent del PIB de Dominicana en 2016, según WTTC." *Diario Turístico de la República Dominicana* (Santo Domingo, DR), March 22, 2017.

Vargas, Joan. "La República Dominicana ocupa cuarto lugar en trabajo sexual." *El Día* (Santo Domingo, DR), Nov. 30, 2017.

Yakushko, Oksana, Manijeh Badiee, Anitra Mallory, and Sherry Wang. "Insider Outsider: Reflections on Working with one's own communities." *Women & Therapy* 34, no. 3 (2011): 279–292.

Chapter Three

Making a Man

Reflections on Masculinities and Bodily Capital in the Chongos *of Quito, Ecuador*

Ronnie Anthony Shepard and Tia Tyndal

It was a cool summer night when I made my return to Quito to conduct fieldwork. On Tuesday, just a few days after my arrival, León extended an invitation to go out and catch up. As we drove through the city, he asked, "Where do you want to go?" I hadn't spoken Spanish in some time and was still unwittingly switching back and forth between languages. "Why don't we go to a nightclub?" I asked, and he agreed. We quickly arrived at a dark building that I had never noticed on any of my prior visits to the city, with only a few red lights illuminating a single window. Upon leaving the car, there was no music to be heard coming from the building or the immediate vicinity. "Where are we?" I asked, and he told me a nightclub. Confused, I asked if he was sure. He confirmed that we were, in fact, at the right place, and proceeded to rattle off a list of prices for different sexual services. It was only then that I realized that "nightclub" means something very different in Ecuador than it does in the United States. There would be no dancing at this nightclub; we were standing in the front door of a local brothel.

This somewhat humorous situation is indicative of the role that commercial sex plays in the creation of Latin American masculine identities. In this chapter, we position the heterosexual sex trade in Quito within the framework of masculinities proposed by anthropologist Xavier Andrade. In his edited volume *Masculinidades en el Ecuador* (2001), Andrade posits that there are five relevant themes that must be addressed when discussing the formation of masculine identities in Latin America: questions of fatherhood; change and resistance to change in the dominant conceptions of masculinity; the racialization of the masculine; machismo and politics; and the paradox of the excess and the silence in the language about bodies and sexuality. Using interstitial excerpts from fieldnotes collected by Ronnie

Shepard in Quito over several years, we argue that these themes mean there is more to sex work than a simple business transaction between consenting individuals; the gender-role socialization included in such interactions cannot be ignored. However, make no mistake, this chapter is not about prostitution or sex work; it is a chapter about the role that culturally defined sex work often plays in "making men."

METHODS

Intrigued by the casualness with which my friend brought me to the nightclub, I began to question León about how common it was for men to visit these places. I was told it was normal for men to go both in groups and individually, although it is not casually discussed with women. He then proceeded to show me four other brothels in the immediate area, and I started to believe that commercial sex in the country is even more common than I initially suspected.

Participant observation for this investigation, including visits to several significant brothels in Quito, was conducted by Shepard with the invaluable assistance of three informants and their network of close friends and family, and several interactions are highlighted throughout. This leads to the anthropologist's own experiences playing an integral role in the study and, as such, necessitates insertion into the narrative. The resultant data was shared with co-author, Tia Tyndal.

In addition to participant observation, we delved into the existing research on men that engage in the commercial sex trade and found that historically, the focus has typically been on either sex workers' experiences or an attempt at characterizing the clients that purchase sex. For a system that has existed for millennia, there is a lack of contextual and developmental analysis on its role in culturally-defined masculinities. Additionally, much of the research has taken place in white-dominated Western societies, which negates the need to incorporate cultural factors exclusive to subaltern populations into the equation. Through many of the dominant research lenses, research has often failed to critically analyze the role that the commercial sex trade plays in creating and maintaining subaltern narratives of masculinity.

Although the performances and definitions of masculinities differ based on locations, cultures, and societies, some of the archetypal features of masculinity in the sexual sphere are that heterosexual men are sexually desirable, experienced, sexually skilled, and have the power to access women of their choosing (Barker and Ricardo 2005). For many men that do not have the realistic ability or access to reach this standard, the commercial sex trade allows them a medium through which masculinities become attainable. Therefore it quickly becomes a defining marker in entering manhood. This may explain why prior research that focuses on men who purchase sex find that these men often do not deviate very far from the norm (Holzman and Pines 1982; Pitts et al. 2004). The investigation presented in this chapter also endorses this finding, and it shows that the males who participate in commercial sex are not inherently "bad" or "criminal"; they are men that we would realistically encounter throughout our daily lives, despite these traditional stereotypes. As a means of exploring beyond the transactional nature of commercial sex and into the personal lives of the men involved while protecting them from said stereotypes, there is a need to maintain a level of anonymity.

Because of the questionable nature regarding the legalities and regulation of the commercial sex industry in Ecuador, the names of any informants questioned in the study have been changed and members of their network generalized. The three most prominent informants of the study are:

> León—male, twenty-five years old, upper-middle class. León is the son of a doctor, yet resides in a working-class sector of the city. He is currently in a committed, monogamous relationship. León is a first-year graduate student in business at a well-regarded university, and a manager in his family's chain of pharmacies marketed to the working class. He lives at home with his parents and his brother, Pol.
>
> Pol—male, twenty-three years old, upper-middle class. Pol is the younger brother of León. Although he has a "girlfriend" who believes they are in a monogamous, committed relationship, he sees several women casually and does not consider himself committed. He is also the father of a three-year-old daughter from a prior relationship. After spending time in a pre-med program, Pol took time off from school and is currently a second-year undergraduate student in gastronomy. He works sporadically, and during the course of this study he held at least three different jobs.
>
> Alexa—twenty-two, female, upper-middle class. Alexa was León's girlfriend, and at the beginning of the study they had been in a committed, monogamous relationship for approximately one year. As a graduate student, she has a permanent job in a male-dominated field already in place upon completion of her degree. Alexa lives at home with her family on a private street in an upper-class sector of Quito.

Although this chapter considers larger themes of masculine identity in Quito, the individual experiences shared by the informants are not meant to be representative of all men in the city. Instead, they are intended to be examples of the ways commercial sex has affected the formation of identity in this specific network. When initially questioned about brothels in the city, women regularly reacted with a hint of disgust, with Alexa referring to the sex workers as "pigs." The reaction of each of the men when broached with the subject of prostitution or upon mention of the nightclub incident was always the same: "Let's go to a *chongo*!"[1]

MACHISMO AS MISNOMER

Masculinity in Latin America is often oversimplified to one word: *machismo*. Machismo has often become a catch-all to address and explain any negative descriptors related to Latin American men, no matter how misguided. While it is true that the idea of machismo is related to masculinity, it is only one small part of larger socially constructed masculinities. In his edited volume *Changing Men and Masculinities in Latin America* (2003), Matthew Gutmann tells us that the term "masculinity" and the related concepts of male identity, manhood, manliness, and men's roles can be defined in four distinct ways, although they often intersect. He says:

> The first concept of *masculinity* argues that it is anything that men think, say and do. If men are involved, then so too must be masculinity. The second holds that masculinity is what men think or say or do to distinguish themselves as men. Accordingly, men may achieve (or strive to achieve) masculinity at sometimes more than at others. Third, masculinity is seen by some as a quality that certain men have more than other men, either because they were born that way, or because of some kind of personal achievement. Finally, other scholars of men and masculinities in Latin America have sought to emphasize the overriding significance of women to the negotiation of masculinities for most if not all men at most if not all times in their lives.

Andrade recognizes Gutmann's description of masculinity in his own work in the field. He acknowledges that the most significant work has been done by Gutmann and Mara Viveros Vigoya, and uses their prior work in his discussion of the five relevant themes of masculinity. Much as there is no overarching idea of Latin American machismo, there is also no overarching Latin American masculine identity. What is considered masculine can often vary by region, country, or even by city. Andrade recognizes this and applies an Ecuadorean lens to his five themes of masculinity, the first of which is fatherhood.

FATHERHOOD AS MASCULINE IDENTITY

In her work "Reflections on Machismo in Latin America," Norma Fuller explains, "the ability to start a family and protect them from other males are the ideals of masculinity" (1998, 261). This meaning supplants an earlier period of youth characterized by an emphasis on sexual performance and virility. Fuller describes this as a period "in which the male must prove that he is sexually active and strong in front of his peers," and only through this period can a male achieve "the true masculinity" (261). This is where the *chongos* come in.

The willingness of all the male informants in this study to go to a chongo as a group characterizes Fuller's period of sexual performance on the road to adulthood. While it is true that older men, both single as well as married, may also solicit the services of sex workers, it is this earlier period of youth that contributes to the formation of masculinities. Three of the males in this network had girlfriends at the time, with relationships ranging in time from one month to five years. When questioned about their eagerness to go to a chongo, they all professed that they love their girlfriends, along with differing variations of "It's OK; we're guys." These variations were all followed up with requests that nothing be said about it to their girlfriends. This showcases the compartmentalization that men must engage in to maintain both their public relationships and private sexual lives without seeing the two as direct contradictions. Clearly, their participation in the commercial sex trade did not come from a place of necessity but instead a place of excess or choice that they wanted to maintain.

Although virginity in potential mates did not seem to be as necessary in this study as it may be in studies of other communities in Latin America, it was assumed by the men in this social network that females would not have as much sexual experience as males. In Gloria Gonzalez-Lopez's study of Mexican immigrants and their sex lives in Los Angeles, she cites Dennis Altman, saying, "Gender and sexuality come together through the family, and family structures themselves, far from being fixed or 'natural' as moral conservatives insist, are ultimately dependent on social and economic structures." (Gonzalez-Lopez 2005, 7) We see this statement proven time and again through the recollections of her subjects and the changes that are made within their lives depending on the proximity to their families. Among the subjects of the Gonzalez-Lopez study, family and sexuality go hand in hand, and the public nature of their ties influences the subjects' sex lives. Proximity to the family has an influence in Ecuador, as well. Consider this note on Pol and his thoughts on relationships while still living at home with his family, particularly his mother:

> *Pol would not consider a "serious" relationship with another woman as long as he lived at home with his parents, preferring to go to a chongo instead. He had lived on his own at various times but had also moved back home on more than one occasion. His mother expected him to be with the mother of his child as a*

> *family. He explained, "My mother will never accept me with anyone else. She hates any other girl I date. She says I need to be a man and be with my family. I rather just go to a chongo and not worry about it."*

In this sense, masculinity is a negotiated process in which the male is being defined both as a family man and as a consumer of commercial sex. This also falls in line with the popular "no-strings-attached" narrative seen in many studies, where men often find sex with sex workers as desirable because it frees them of the obligations associated with romantic relationships and guarantees them sex through a simple transaction (Huysamen and Boonzaier 2014).

In speaking with Pol's mother privately, she validated his previously expressed concerns. In conversation, the subject of fatherhood was broached, albeit unintentionally. After inquiring as to the reasons why Shepard was not married and a father at his age, his mother began to speak about Pol and his relationship with his daughter. Teary-eyed, she divulged:

> *Every night I pray that he will go back to his wife and be a good father. A child needs a father in their life. I keep waiting, and he still won't be responsible. This is going to damage her (the daughter) as she grows up. It's not good for her father not to be there.*

The respondent's mother is not only preaching familial responsibility to her son, but she is also perpetuating patriarchal norms that have lasted for centuries, as well as notions of masculinity and what is perceived to be a "real man." Modernity is colliding with beliefs that have extended to at least the colonial era and the arrival of Spanish forces. In the words of Charles Goolsby, Jr. (2003), "The imposition of Roman and later Moorish conquests on Spain imported common Mediterranean attitudes of women as the property of men, to be guided, controlled and limited in their freedom throughout life by fathers, brothers, and husbands." Today, according to Fuller, the similarity of experiences between young males in Mediterranean societies and the period of young adulthood characterized by sexual conquests in Latin American males can be understood as "characteristic features of a moment in the life of men in patriarchal societies with sharply divided male and female spheres" (Fuller 1998, 259). Still, it is through both maturity and the proving of their virility that young men in Ecuador and across the region can reach fatherhood as a viable masculine identity.

Fatherhood as an identity is in a period of transition. With modernity have come changing attitudes towards both child rearing and gender roles. These changes are by no means homogeneous, with Viveros Vigoya noting that there is a "great variability in the experience of fatherhood according to men's socioeconomic and ethnic-racial allegiances, their generations, their primary experiences, specific moments of the life cycles in which they find themselves, and the sexes and ages of their children" (2003, 42). This can be seen in Pol's familial relationships. While he spends little time with his three-year-old daughter, his upper-class father took his granddaughter several days of the week. On days that the child spent the night, she always slept in the room with her grandparents. The grandfather also enjoyed a good relationship with his two sons, playing on the same local *fútbol* team and sharing the ability to talk about relationships that was off-limits to his wife.

CHANGE AND RESISTANCE TO CHANGE IN THE DOMINANT CONCEPTIONS OF MASCULINITY

Andrade's second masculine identity of note is that of change and resistance to change in the dominant conceptions of masculinity. He makes clear that the dominant conceptions in Ecuador are those of homosociality, discipline, and vengeance. These ideas are tied into the public performance of masculinity. We focus here on the primary conception—that of homosociality—while also considering to a lesser extent the following two.

Homosociality

Denise Jardim argues that in Latin America it is important for men to be able to share moments with other men to reflect on ideal masculine behavior. Witness this contest of one-upmanship between two heterosexual males in a homosocial space in Quito. This took place in a gender-specific steam room shortly after Shepard had been introduced to both men. The first is the twenty-three-year-old son of a diplomat from the Middle East and his Ecuadorean wife (A). The second is his nineteen-year-old and locally born working-class friend and classmate (B). The entire interaction took place before Shepard was able to respond:

A: "Ronnie, es gay."	Ronnie, he is gay.
B: "¡Y él es mi pareja!"	And he is my boyfriend!
A: "Sí, pero es la mujer en la relación."	Yes, but he's the woman in the relationship.

While both men self-identified as heterosexual, the intended goal was clear: by challenging the inherent manhood of each other, the respondents were asserting their own manliness among other men. This verbal jousting was followed up by laughter from the whole group, and there were no hard feelings between the two individuals involved. The exchange is not dissimilar to Andrade's study of *homosocialidad* in Guayaquil, Ecuador, in which two of his informants, members of a network of young men from a local barrio, spent an evening competing not through words, but by vying for the traditionally male role in a couples' dance (Andrade 2001a). Viveros Vigoya, in quoting Jardim, would argue that the steam room itself acts as a "privileged space for male socialization in which discourse about the meanings of being male are produced and reproduced." (Viveros Vigoya 2003, 43) In fact, many upscale apartment buildings throughout Ecuador have gender-specific steam rooms for men only. When they create these social spaces for males—either institutionally dictated or culturally understood and accepted—and do not create similar gender-specific areas dedicated to women, we see an example of hegemonic patriarchal ideas being built directly into the architecture of the country. Vastly different beliefs and the resultant stigma surrounding commercial sex in many countries would make many men reluctant to share the details of their participation in homosocial (and heterosocial) spaces. In Ecuador, men may gain credit or validation of their masculinity through sharing these experiences with other men.

The group experience of visiting a chongo may in fact be a high-water mark in the public performance of masculinity, as now the male must not only boast about his sexual prowess and experiences but is now also expected to perform in a sexual way. Bernstein would argue that this illustrates a time where "technically illegal commercial sex acts are consumed as relatively unproblematic instances of sexual entitlement and male bonding." Still, as previously mentioned it is an experience toward forming identity that can be shared among the group. It also gives the male an opportunity to have sexual experiences that may be more highly favored by both the individual as well as the group. This may present itself as experiences with women who have migrated from other parts of the country or internationally. Race and ethnicity regularly play a role in the selection of partners, and both have a monetary impact on transactions in the chongos. This is further explored in a subsequent section of this chapter, "Race and the Masculine."

Discipline

In *Masculinidades en Ecuador*, Andrade recounts the story of a gender-ambiguous person he encounters on a bus heading from Guayaquil to Salitre, an area perceived as "the most violent society on the Ecuadorean coast," yet, almost ironically, he is assured, "that homosexuality is very well tolerated and appears to be displayed publicly without much fuss, at least under festive circumstances" (Andrade 2001, 123). Upon seeing the person, Andrade is surprised—a result of conditioning to expect the dominant heterosexual norms, a male/female dichotomy "with positive signs of naturalness, exclusivity, and domination" whose visual cues cause the viewer to think "masculine" and feminine" (Andrade 2001a, 124). Kowtowing to these dominant representations of gender identity in order to preserve the heteronormative status quo often results in attempts at "passing," due to "understanding sexuality as a dimension of power (that intersects with other dimensions such as race, gender, and class) in which certain groups are privileged over others," in this case, the heterosexual (Cantú 2003, 271). The passenger on Andrade's bus, while treated as simply "one of the girls" by the two women accompanying him/her, challenged the masculine ideals of sexual and gender discipline in the subtlest of ways: by just wearing a small earring and some eyeliner hidden by sunglasses, yet retaining a short hairstyle and men's clothing, he/she emphasized some semblance of a woman yet could not easily be considered a transvestite. In terms of gender "performance," Andrade encounters a conundrum; he believes "he was more likely to be seen as a gay male with emphasized feminine traits, but her performance to her friends was of 'passing' as just one of them."[2] It was only when the bus reached a makeshift checkpoint and a local militia ordered all of the men to step off the bus to be frisked that he registered that his gender took precedence over the image that was presented. The officer charged with the responsibility of frisking asserted his masculinity by feigning disgust and acting as if the passenger were contagious. It was only through the quick intervention of the passenger's female friends dancing inside the bus and acting flirtatious with the officer, thus reaffirming his inherent manliness, that the male travelers were once again allowed to board, and the bus at last was allowed to continue to its destination.

Andrade recognizes that there are stereotypical images applied to both Guayaquil and Quito, saying that "Guayaquil, according to representations of Quito associated with regionalism, is characterized as having a 'more *machista* (macho)' culture than the capital." He challenges this myth by declaring, "contrary to this stereotype, daily observations in the center of Guayaquil reveal the quotidian appropriation of fragments of this space, such as the renovated Centennial Park, by members of informal groups of transvestites and male homosexual strata, despite the strong stigma held against such sexualities" (Andrade 2001, 123). In turn, challenging the image of Quito as more tolerant of sexual dissidents is this anecdote from the fieldnotes of an incident witnessed during Shepard's night in the chongos, with the entirety of the night discussed in greater detail later in the chapter:

> *As I was in the car with León and Alexa traveling from one brothel to the next, we came across a scene involving the police and several transvestite sex workers. We quickly pulled on to a side street and parked the car in order to watch*

what was taking place. It appeared as if the police officers were simply amusing themselves through harassment and intimidation. After several long minutes of back-and-forth antagonism between the opposing groups, the transvestites finally offered their IDs to the police for inspection. After looking over the IDs, the officers gave each other a little laugh before handing them back. The workers were defiant to the end, yelling at the officers even as they got back into their car to leave.

It should be highlighted that for those born biologically male in both Guayaquil and Quito the simple act of dressing in female clothing while male is itself a socially transgressive act regularly subject to, at best, public scrutinization, and at worst, violence. Truly, "civic discipline, and the form of masculinity that this implies, is a contested process" (Andrade 2001a, 126).

Vengeance

Theoretical notions of vengeance as a signifier of masculine identity are more difficult to ascertain, with Andrade having to use a scene from Hugo Idrovo's musical *La Saga y el Gozo* to illustrate his point. In the scene, titled "La Esquina" (The Corner), the main character discovers his girlfriend is having a sexual affair with a man outside of the relationship—a black man. With several mentions of the man's race, and, in turn, the size of his phallus, the main character feels his only recourse is to kill his rival for the woman's affections. He kills the man on a local street corner in front of several witnesses including his girlfriend, with his final revenge being to sever the man's penis, displaying it for the entire neighborhood to see. Even though the man is dead, this symbolic assertion of dominant masculinity and the emasculation of his rival is significant, as "the phallus is master-signifier, and femininity is symbolically defined as lack" (Connell 2005, 70). In retaliation for this murder, the main character is killed as well—on the very corner the initial murder took place.

The main character's need for vengeance is fueled by two points: Firstly, his girlfriend chose as her lover an *esmeraldeño*, symbolically a black man, and, stereotypically, a man of great sexual prowess and phallic size. Connell would note this is problematic because "white men's masculinities are constructed not only in relation to white women but also in relation to black men" (2005, 75). Secondly, the man had a reputation as "a talker, someone who likes to surround himself with exaggerations and lies, presumably including those relating to his own masculinity" (Andrade 2001, 129).

The character's public vindication comes in four stages of public performance: by acts of bravado in front of other men, by performing revenge against his rival, by displaying the castrated phallus in front of his girlfriend, and finally, by losing his own life in a public display. Andrade states that for the main character, "the public performance of acts of bravado, revenge, disputes, and killing served as a framework for material actions leading to castration and death" (2001a, 129). With the circulation and consumption of masculinity a constant through successive displays of the male body throughout the play, castration and death become carefully considered displays of what is considered truly "male," and vengeance becomes a manifestation of true masculinity.

One could also argue that some of the violence seen directed at sex workers within the commercial sex trade may fall into this category. Men, when confronted with emasculation, may resort to high hostility/sexual aggression to over-perform masculinity. Farley et al. (2017) found that men who purchase sex had greater hostile masculinity as well as a greater history for sexual aggression. Vengeance within the commercial sex trade may showcase itself as various forms of violence against sex workers.

RACE AND THE MASCULINE

Much has been written about the whitening and/or darkening of races to create ideal traits. Marisol de la Cadena's (2000) analysis of the initial whitening and subsequent feminization of the white male to create a national identity in neighboring Peru is a prime example. Work on the erotic symbolism of women in the Andes has also had its share of work. The physical attributes of the women involved in the commerce of sex is integral for both the men and the women. For the men, the opportunity for bragging rights presents itself in the form of experiences with women that may be particularly valued in their social spheres. The physicality of the women in turn becomes bodily capital, that "symbolic currency often acquired by members of the dominated fractions of society, who, deprived of other forms of social power, cultivate their bodies as value-producing investments" (Bernstein 2007, 42). This leads to men becoming ethno-adventurers, or "the undertakers of sexual expeditions across ethnic divides for recreational, casual or 'exotic' encounters, often more than once, but returning to their sexual home bases after each excursion" (Nagel 2003, 14). The brothel itself is an ethnosexual frontier, those supervised, regulated, and restricted erotic locations and destinations where individuals regularly forge sexual links with ethnic Others.

For the network of men in this study, women who had migrated from the Ecuadorean city of Chone and Colombian women were particularly prized as they were perceived to be more curvaceous. León, putting it more succinctly, shared, "*En América Latina, si no hay culo que no hay nada.* (In

Latin America, if there's no ass, there's nothing)." Conversely, native Indian women and women of African descent are regularly devalued. Anglo women from both the United States and Europe were prized as well, albeit for a different reason: the color of their skin. Curious of the way men in the network fawned over any Anglo women they saw, Shepard asked one of the men, a twenty-seven-year-old with darker skin than the other men in the group. His response given with a laugh was simply, "In Ecuador we have a saying: '*Para el mejoramiento de la raza*. (For the betterment of the race.)'" This illustrates that race not only plays a significant role in Ecuadorean society, as it does in most places, but in masculinities and sexualities, as well.

To further expound on this discourse of race and the eroticization of ethnic "Others," consider this account of the familial makeup of two informants. The father of the family is an ex-diplomat who was stationed in Ecuador. He met and started a family with a brown-skinned Ecuadorean woman which includes two sons included in this network: a twenty-three-year-old student (mentioned previously in this chapter), and his twenty-nine-year-old brother. This brother, in turn, had a son with a light-skinned Ecuadorean woman. He ended the relationship when he met a fair-skinned German woman. They have been in a committed relationship for five years. He still visits the chongos, most frequently when his girlfriend is not in town. His father, he attests, has visited them, as well.

Of the brothels discussed during fieldwork, the network agreed that those with Colombian women charged higher rates for their services. The men in the group considered the higher cost worth it. The dramatic differences in what Shepard calls "racialized rates" becomes abundantly clear during his night in the chongos, discussed in detail later in this chapter.

MACHISMO AND POLITICS

In the summer of 1999, the entire province of Guayas, including Guayaquil, Ecuador, was under an imposed state of martial law. This state of emergency was heralded by the political and economic elites (i.e., the holders of hegemonic masculinity) in the city. It was during this politically based state of terror that Andrade's encounter with the gender-ambiguous bus passenger took place. Andrade uses the climate of fear in this period to illustrate that masculine rhetoric is often employed by the state. He says, "The dominant language used by the authorities and media elites is that of war, a male language par excellence: 'fight until all the bad people, the criminals, are subject to the order of the State,' 'defend the rights of honest citizens' have been loaded phrases of masculine heroism" (Andrade 2001a, 122).

The masculinity of the state can be put into action, as well. By ordering the men off the bus and frisked, backs to the officers, the State constructed a form of emasculation while also promoting its own masculine imagery. The visual inspection of the passengers' IDs, much like Shepard's recollection of the heated encounter between transvestite sex workers and the police, only adds to the perceived supremacy of the State and its oppression of the citizenry, as now the State is also controlling representations of identity.

In his discussion of the contested and fluctuating meanings of the words *macho* and *machismo* in Mexico, Gutmann's study of Mexican masculinities shares a great deal of similarity with Andrade's theories on the Ecuadorean State. Gutmann affirms that while society as a whole can be considered *macho*, it is still important to consider definitions and contexts. Clarifying, he shares, "In financial and government circles, in the arts, the universities, and the media, men predominate and dominate. In terms of who rules Mexican society and its central institutions, the issue is so straightforward that male domination there is a classic example of hegemonic, taken-for-granted control" (Gutmann 2007, 237). Further illuminating the state as a masculine institution, Connell declares that "state organizational practices are structured in relation to the reproductive arena. The overwhelming majority of top office-holders are men because there is a gender configuring of recruitment and promotion, a gender configuring of the internal division of labor and systems of control, a gender configuring of policymaking, practical routines, and ways of mobilizing pleasure and consent" (Connell 2005, 73).

There is a vested political interest in the chongos of Ecuador, with influence ranging from international mafias to political elites. Because of these ties, prosecution of all types (taxes, human trafficking, rape, etc.) is extremely limited. Politicians and high-ranking officials are often patrons of the establishments, hindering the desire for prosecution even further. Particularly favored among elites is a chongo called The Doll House, which will be further discussed.

CONSIDERING BODIES AND SEXUALITY

The environment within homosocial spaces is undoubtedly sexually charged, with talk of sex a constant during conversation. This may take the form of discussing "sexual conquests," discussions of women and their bodies, or general name-calling. Yet for all the braggadocio, there is little actual discourse among men about bodies and/or the female form. Consider these two separate awkward conversations, one slightly embarrassing, the other slightly astonishing, with men included in the network of informants. From the fieldnotes:

Today I walked through La Mariscal with Pol. I noticed that a restaurant named G-Spot had painted over its signage and outer walls since the last time I had been in Quito, yet the name had not changed. This led to a conversation about the varying meanings of the term "G-Spot." I assumed he knew that for the tourists coming from the United States, the name and the stylized white splatter-marks of paint used to decorate the outside of the restaurant connoted its more sexual overtones. He insisted a G-Spot was a nickname for one thousand dollars. This led to a deluge of questions regarding what a G-Spot is and where it is located on a woman, with Pol finally accepting that it is not a vagina and deciding that it was equivalent to punto-g, *a term since adopted as the name of a dance club in the city.*

The second conversation took place with Pol and his "girlfriend":

Today the topic of HIV/AIDS came up, and Pol stated, matter-of-factly, "If you get it, you're dead." I explained to him that this was not the case and tried my best to explain the use of anti-retroviral medications to help combat the disease. His state of bewilderment at this was matched by my own awe at his unknowing, as his father is a doctor, and his family runs a chain of pharmacies in which he used to work (his brother and pharmacy manager León, it should be noted, was fully aware of the disease and its treatments).

This lack of awareness is seen in much of the research focused on men who engage in the commercial sex trade. Themes arise when analyzing prevalent intents for the sexual encounter. Some of these themes include the belief that the women are "pros" with exceptional sexual powers that are willing to provide special services, as well as the belief that the man could seduce the woman into desiring him by being pleasant or amorous, resulting in a more energetic participant (Holzman and Pines 1982). Intimacy is also commonly seen as a theme, with men expecting the woman to provide above and beyond the physical sexual service to include intimacy, as well, so that the experience bears a resemblance to a real romantic encounter (Huysamen and Boonzaier 2014). The sex trade then provides a context where men can perform an idealized form of male heterosexuality while remaining ignorant of actual bodies and sexuality.

The ignorance, while unfortunate, can also be dangerous due to the increased risk of health-related concerns. On average men who purchase sex have significantly more lifetime partners than men who do not (Farley et al. 2017). An increase in sexual partners often increases the risk of sexually transmitted infections (STIs). In addition, a lack of condom use is often seen among male clients. Gertler and Shah (2010) found that 23 percent of sex workers reported experiencing some type of STI in the last year and 52 percent reported ever having had an STI, which is a much higher STI rate than that of the general population. They attribute this to low condom use and untreated STIs, which are conditions that also make it easier for the transmission of the HIV virus. The UN-AIDS report (2002) lists unprotected sex with sex workers as making up a large portion of the approximately 20,000 people who acquire HIV each day (Gertler and Shah 2010).

In recent years, scholars have called for a closer look at male involvement in the realm of reproduction, a realm traditionally devoted to women. Viveros Vigoya (2003) theorizes that by calling attention to male behavior and attitudes towards sexual and reproductive health in their own right and from male points of view in various cultural contexts it would be possible to "construct new models of family life and gender relations on a more democratic and equal basis throughout the region" (47). Gutmann recognizes this call to action and highlights the work of feminist scholars, saying "fortunately indeed, many feminist theories of gender inequality help provide the framework within which we are today able to develop the contrasting study of men, sexuality, reproduction, and masculinity as integral to a more general project of exploring the history and diversity of gender/sexuality systems in the world" (2007, 29).

Although the commercial sex trade is not technically legal in Ecuador (the informants thought differently), it is both tolerated and regulated by the state, essentially giving men power over the female body. According to journalist Dominique Soguel (2009), "Brothels derive their legitimacy not from the law but from a series of health and sanitation certificates from local health authorities that add up to 'centers of tolerance,' where prostitution is accepted." The sex workers in the brothels are required to be tested on a weekly basis and are given health cards that are then shown to potential clients upon request. On the surface, it appears to be working: even though the Ministry of Health reports that the country's HIV-AIDS infection rate more than doubled between 2004 and 2007, with 80 percent linked to heterosexual activity; in all cases reported in 2007 only one was linked to a female sex worker. These statistics may not be accurate, as the Ministry of Health only monitors licensed venues, and unlicensed brothels are numerous. Women and minors are often also smuggled into the country, tricked by men through the promise of high-paying jobs and instead forced into indentured servitude and hidden from sight, making actual numbers difficult to ascertain. The role of women in the brothels themselves is quite restricted; in some, upon payment for sexual activity—which is given to men working in the brothels as opposed to the women performing the actual acts—the man is given an alcoholic beverage, (there is almost always a drink minimum) as well as a condom, which is often also provided by a male employee. This mirrors the traditional heterosexual scripts that portray women as the boundary setters and gatekeepers of their bodies, while men must offer something in exchange for access (Seal and Ehrhardt 2003), but instead empowers men to make the rules and play the game, effectively cutting women out of the interaction.

A NIGHT IN THE CHONGOS: UNCOVERING MANHOOD IN THE BROTHELS OF QUITO

Tonight, I set off on a solo journey to explore life in the brothels of Quito. My initial foray was before sundown. As I walked through La Mariscal, the area of the city often referred to by locals as "Gringolándia" *due to its consistently high concentration of tourists, I looked for the telltale red lights signifying commercial sex. I did not have to look far; instead, it was the sex industry that found me.*

As I walked towards Plaza Foch, a plaza in La Mariscal centered directly in the heart of Quito's nightlife, I heard a woman's voice calling down to me from the second floor of a building I had previously known only as a karaoke bar. This came as a surprise to me. Although it is all too common to hear cat calls shouted down to women from men in buildings or construction sites, this bit of gendered role-reversal caught me off-guard. I looked up to find a woman dressed in a negligee, hanging seductively out of a window. As she caught my attention, our verbal interaction was brief: "Are you American?" she asked. "Yes," I responded.

With this confirmation, the woman allowed one of the straps to slide off her shoulder, fully aware of the ways to use her body as a form of capital. After overcoming my initial shock and having noticed the tourists starting to stare back and forth between me and her breast, I hurriedly walked off, deciding to continue my exploration of males in the brothels that night.

Ecuador's chongos are marketed to potential clientele based on race and ethnicity, age, and social class. To take the investigation full circle, arrangements were made with León, who unwittingly brought Shepard to his first brothel, to visit as many chongos as possible in one evening. His girlfriend Alexa insisted on joining in. A concerted effort was made to visit chongos popular with men of different classes. When moving from location to location, León and Alexa shared some of the behind-the-scenes information that cannot be gleaned by simply entering and observing. This was also the last opportunity to question the two about their thoughts on men and brothels. Although Alexa was unwilling to enter the brothels, saying curiously, "I'm not friends with those people," she proved more than willing to take pictures outside and was surprisingly non-judgmental in discussing what takes place inside. To keep repetition to a minimum, we have chosen to discuss only the four most well-known sites below. In this section of the chapter, Shepard describes what he saw and some of the interactions inside, and those with León and Alexa. Conversations between the three were recorded using a hand-held voice recorder and select portions have been translated and included here.

Kasandra

Kasandra is jokingly referred to by *quiteños*[3] as K.F.C. Playing on the abbreviation for Kentucky Fried Chicken, it acts in this case as a crass abbreviation for "Kasandra Fucking Club" or "Kasandra Full Culeo," depending on who is asked. The chongo is located on La Panamericana Norte, a major thoroughfare in an area dotted with warehouses.[4] The area was formerly a red-light district, and at one point each of the warehouses was part of Kasandra. The entire area has since been converted into an industrial zone, leaving only Kasandra's current location, with the sex workers from the others relocated to other sites throughout the city. Of all the chongos located in Quito, Kasandra is one of the most well known, and arguably, due to its low rates and women from both Colombia and the Ecuadorean coast, one of its most popular.

The outside of Kasandra looks less like a brothel and more like the surrounding industrial zone. There is a large wall blocking the view from the outside and a large metal sliding door which is opened by security guards, allowing you to drive inside. The grounds behind the gate are covered in haphazardly parked cars. The inside looks like a large disco with many women surrounding the bar. Exotic dancers also perform in this area, both solo and in groups. I was approached by an employee, a male, who informed me that the cost was ten dollars for an hour with an Ecuadorean woman, and twenty-five dollars with a Colombian. León thought this was too much and probably due to my status as a United States citizen. Either way, I respectfully declined.

Kasandra, located in the northern part of Quito, caters to men of the lower and middle classes.

515

For upper-class men only, 515 is located across the street from another upper-class brothel called Cinco Estrellas,[5] and across the parking lot from a children's toy store. There is an extremely high door fee just to get inside, with prices continuing from there. Here, León describes the financial intricacies of what takes place inside:

> What happens is the men here receive their paychecks, or their salary, and they want to spend it on *putas* (whores). Imagine, a mason that receives the minimum salary, two hundred twenty dollars, he goes to Kasandra and spends the whole night. Here, a bottle of whiskey costs you a hundred dollars. Sex is another one

> hundred twenty dollars. In contrast, in Kasandra it's an even twenty dollars to have sex with the *putas*, or per *ficha* (chip), because all the chongos use *fichas* to enter a room. Here, you pay one hundred dollars just to get inside.

Fully aware of the status of racialized rates at Kasandra from my visit there, I decided to press León further on some of the costs associated with commercial sex at 515. He continued:

> There are different prices depending on the *puta*. If she is Colombian, if she is hot, she costs more. There are also tariffs for each sex act. If you only want oral sex it goes down a little, but there is always a tariff.

The owners of 515 are fully aware of their desired clientele and specifically situated the chongo in a well-off area of the city, where it is surrounded by professional organizations devoted to fields like architecture, medicine, and engineering. As we stood outside, the doors opened as the doormen were letting patrons out. Alexa attempted to take pictures of this, but the doormen saw us. León quickly snatched the camera out of her hands, and we hurriedly headed to the next destination, with Alexa noting that even the cars in the parking lot were of a higher class than those seen at Kasandra.

4033

Another popular chongo, albeit for different reasons, is 4033. Located directly across the street from another brothel called Tango Cache, 4033 is most popular among young men still in high school or those that have recently entered college, as the doormen do not ask for identification in order to enter. The brothel is unique in that it is also a branch. As León explains, "This chongo has a branch, another chongo with the same name below Universidad U.T.E. There are two, and they both have the same owner." He further divulged that he had not been there in several years, as he believes the chongo caters to men between fifteen and twenty years old. It appears that the owner is fully aware of his clientele, as well, as he has located both branches of 4033 within short walking distance of universities. In terms of name recognition, León argues that 4033 is at least on a par with Kasandra.

It should be noted that throughout our journey from chongo to chongo, León spoke without trepidation about the chongos he has visited and what he knew of others, with Alexa present. She, in turn, chimed in whenever she felt she had knowledge to contribute. This level of comfort and familiarity was replicated whenever I spoke about brothels among mixed groups of men and women. The only point in which León and Alexa disagreed was when I broached the subject of married men and commercial sex. As we left 4033 and headed to the next location, the dialogue went as follows:

Ronnie: In Ecuador, is it normal for husbands to go to the chongos?

León (with Alexa): Yes.

Alexa (with León): No.

A: Depends. No, no, no.

L: In general, yes.

A: No! Husbands that are whores, yes. The decent ones, no.

L: In general, yes. Eighty percent of married men frequent the chongos.

A: No! You are such a whore!

While León's thoughts on the frequency of visits by married men in Ecuador are highly debatable, Alexa's reaction to his statements demonstrates that while she may accept commercial sex as a part of the environment around her, if there is a potential for manifestation in her own life she is not as tolerant. Her refusal to enter any of the establishments works to further illuminate this disassociation.

The Doll House

One of the most famous, most expensive, and perhaps most notorious brothels in all of Ecuador is The Doll House. The brothel is located within walking distance of a *residencia* used by one of the many language schools in the city. Known for its women from Colombia as well as underaged sex workers, the chongo is frequented by diplomats, professional soccer players, foreign tourists, and upper-class Ecuadoreans. On December 10, 2008, in an effort to combat child sex-trafficking and sexual slavery, The Doll House was the site of a highly publicized raid, although it was not the first time the establishment was under investigation. During this particular raid, however, ten men were detained, and twenty-six women (twenty-four Colombian, two Ecuadorean) were rescued. Although much attention was paid to the case, León assured me that there were still underaged girls inside, hidden away when the authorities arrive.

Upon arriving at The Doll House and feeling that I could be both legally and ethically compromised by patronizing an establishment where children are being exploited (never mind the moral malaise churning inside), I declined to enter the building, and León understood. Alexa shared that this was where to come for Colombian women (even though we had already been to Kasandra), while León raved about the women inside, saying, "They are much hotter! And better bodies. Much, much, much better!" I suggested this was just his opinion, and he quickly replied, "In the opinion of men! Of many men who have had them." Outside the building, waiting at the doors, were four American men who had come together and were waiting for the guards to let them inside. As we stood next to them, León shared that he considered The Doll House to be on an equal level with 515, but more well known and more popular. As we spoke, an employee came to the door and told the men that several of the girls had been sent to another chongo for the evening and that they should catch a cab and go there to find them. The new location was owned by the same man.

CONCLUSION

From social circles to business negotiations, from the home and into the community, localized ideals of symbolic masculinity such as race, homosociality, and fatherhood are integral parts of Ecuadorean masculine identity. Viveros Vigoya notes that an important dimension of masculine homosociality is its "expression in public spaces, including symbolic spaces of power in which women have traditionally not been present"[6] (2003, 42). With the country's attempts to modernize, there has been both change and resistance to change in the dominant conceptions of masculinity coming from both men and women. She further notes, "Despite the recent increase in encounters between men and women in time and space, often in Latin America there has been a tendency to reproduce relations grounded in hegemonic masculinity, that is, to ignore or subordinate women" (45). Connell would further describe this masculine hegemony as "the configuration of gender practice which embodies the currently accepted problem of the legitimacy of the patriarchy, which guarantees (or is taken to guarantee) the domination of men" (2005, 77). Still, men have yet to take a primary role in the discourse of sexual and reproductive health, with scholars arguing for the construction of new models of family life and gender relations based on equality. As things presently stand, reproduction is still under its more traditional purview: solely the responsibility of women. These quotidian manifestations of gender roles also show us how brothels can be an underlying force in creating locally defined masculinities.

Although the reasons that men turn to sexual commerce vary, we have cited many examples of what Bernstein notes are some of the primary motivations for consumers of commercial sex, such as "desire for sexual variation, sexual access to partners with preferred ages, racialized bodies and specific physiques, the appeal of an 'emotion-free' and clandestine sexual encounter . . . and the thrill of violating taboos" (2007, 117). These thrills often come as a violation of the human rights of others, with women more often than not bearing the brunt of victimization. Since the creation of the Anti-Trafficking Unit of the police in 2003, one hundred and eighty women have been "rescued" as of this writing, yet only fifteen men have been prosecuted. According to the Ombudsman's Office of Quito, in 2007 alone, "there were one hundred and fifty-two allegations of sexual exploitation to the prosecution. However, only four ended in decision processes." The political connections of the men involved in the upper-echelons of the city's commercial sex industry extend to the far reaches of the globe and are well-documented, yet little is done to temper their control over sexual commerce and the bodies of women.

Masculine identities are often in flux; although brothels are found throughout the country, this chapter concentrated on the metropolitan area of Quito as the cultural differences between *costeños* (people from the coast) and *serranos* (people from the mountains) are often great. The veil of machismo that is often applied to the entire Latin American region is in fact just a small piece of more nuanced masculine identity formation, just as commercial sex is just one tool to assert those identities.

NOTES

1. What is known as a nightclub in the United States translates as *discoteca* in Spanish. In Ecuador, a brothel is alternately known as a *nightclub*, *cabaret, púticlub*, *prostíbulo*, or most commonly, a *chongo*.

2. I use masculine pronouns to describe the passenger in the anecdote after using "he/she" only to maintain the terms Andrade uses within the original Spanish. While he uses terms signifying the passenger's biological gender as male, and the passenger was required to get off the bus with other men, Andrade also acknowledges that he was treated as female by the other women and switches the gender of his pronouns mid-sentence. In the chapter, Andrade never asks the passenger how he/she identifies.

3. In Ecuador, as in many locations throughout Latin America, people are often categorized by the cities they live in or the cities of their birth. *Quiteño* describes someone from Quito, *Guayaquileño* for Guayaquil, and so on.

4. Part of the Pan-American Highway system which, save for the Darién Gap between Colombia and Panama, extends from Argentina through fourteen countries of the Americas, including (unofficially) the United States and Canada.

5. Cinco Estrellas was unique in that it was the only brothel that none of my informants had been to, because all deemed it too expensive. From what they have heard from people who have been inside, it is more of an elaborate disco complete with flashing lights, bars, and dance floor. The only difference is that all the women inside are sex workers, with mini-rooms located around the building used for sexual activity.

6. "Doll House, prostíbulo que nunca cierra"

WORKS CITED

Abad, Angelita, Marena Briones, Tatiana Cordero, Rosa Manzo, and Marta Marchán. 2016. "The Association of Autonomous Women Workers, Ecuador: '22nd June.'" In *Global Sex Workers: Rights, Resistance, and Redefinition*, edited by Kamala Kempadoo and Jo Doezema, 172–177. New York: Routledge.

Acién, Estefanía. 2008. "Migrantes y Trabajo Sexual: Estereotipos e Intervención Social." In *Los Retos de la Prostitución: Estigmatización, derechos y respeto*, edited by José Luis Solana, 59–74. Granada: Editorial Comares, S.L.

Andrade, X. 2003. "Pancho Jaime and the Political Uses of Masculinity in Ecuador." *In Changing Men and Masculinities in Latin America*, edited by Matthew C. Gutmann, 281–304. Durham: Duke University Press.

Andrade, Xavier. 2001a. "Homosocialidad, disciplina, y venganza." In *Masculinidades en Ecuador*, edited by X. Andrade and Gioconda Herrera, 115–138. Quito: FLACSO, Sede Ecuador.

———. 2001b. "Introducción Masculinidades en el Ecuador: Contexto y particularidades." In *Masculinidades en Ecuador*, edited by X. Andrade and Gioconda Herrera, 13–26. Quito: FLACSO, Sede Ecuador.

Bader, Michael. 2009. *Male Sexuality: Why Women Don't Understand It—And Men Don't Either*. Lanham: Rowman and Littlefield Publishers, Inc.

Barker, Gary, and Christine Ricardo. 2006. "Young Men and the Construction of Masculinity in Sub-Saharan Africa: Implications for HIV/AIDS, Conflict and Violence." In *The Other Half of Gender: Men's Issues in Development*, edited by Ian Bannon and Maria C. Correia, 159–94. Washington, DC: The World Bank.

Bernstein, Elizabeth. 2007. *Temporarily Yours: Intimacy, Authenticity, and the Commerce of Sex.* Chicago: University of Chicago Press.

Cantú, Lionel. 2003. "Mexican Immigrant Men's Family Experiences." In *Perspectives on Las Américas*, edited by Matthew Gutmann, 245–273. Malden: Blackwell Publishing.

Connell, R.W. 2005. *Masculinities*. Berkeley: University of California Press.

Crain, Mary M. 1996. "The Gendering of Ethnicity in the Ecuadorean Andes: Native Women's Self-Fashioning in the Urban Marketplace." In *Machos, Mistresses, Madonnas*, edited by Marit Melhuus and Kristi Anne Stølen, 134–158. London: Verso.

De la Cadena, Marisol. 2000. *Indigenous Mestizos: The Politics of Race and Culture in Cuzco, Peru 1919–1991*. Durham: Duke University Press.

Di Nicola, Andrea. 2009. *Prostitution and Human Trafficking: Focus on Clients.* New York: Springer.

Farley, Melissa, Jacqueline M. Golding, Emily Schuckman Matthews, Neil M. Malamuth and Laura Jarrett. (2017). "Comparing Sex Buyers With Men Who Do Not Buy Sex: New Data on Prostitution and Trafficking." *Journal of Interpersonal Violence* 32, no. 23 (2017): 3601–3625. doi: 10.1177/0886260515600874.

Fuller, Norma. 1998. "Reflexiones sobre el Machismo en América Latina." *In Masculinidades y equidad de género en América Latina*, edited by Teresa Valdés and José Olavarría, 258–266. Santiago: FLACSO-Chile.

Gertler, Paul and Manisha Shah. (2011). Sex Work and Infection: What's Law Enforcement Got to Do with It? *Journal of Law & Economics* 40, no. 4 (2010): 811–840. doi: 10.1086/661634.

González, Ray. 1996. *Muy Macho: Latino Men Confront Their Manhood*. New York: Anchor Books, Doubleday.

Gonzalez-Lopez, Gloria. 2005. *Erotic Journeys: Mexican Immigrants and Their Sex Lives*. University of California Press.

Goolsby, Jr. Charles M. 2003. "Dynamics of Prostitution and Sex Trafficking from Latin America into the United States." *Childtrafficking.com Digital Library* (2003). www.childtrafficking.com.

Gutmann, Matthew C. 2003. "Introduction: Discarding Manly Dichotomies in Latin America." In *Changing Men and Masculinities in Latin America*, edited by Matthew C. Gutmann, 1–26. Durham: Duke University Press.

———. 2007. *The Meanings of Macho: Being a Man in Mexico City*. Berkeley: University of California Press.

Gutmann, Matthew. 2007. *Fixing Men: Sex, Birth Control, and AIDS in Mexico*. Berkeley: University of California Press.

Herrera, Gioconda and Lily Rodríguez. 2001. "Masculinidad y equidad de género: desafíos para el campo del desarrollo y la salud sexual y reproductiva." In *Masculinidades en Ecuador*, edited by X. Andrade and Gioconda Herrera, 157–178. Quito: FLACSO, Sede Ecuador.

Holzman, Harold R., and Sharon Pines. 1982. "Buying sex: The phenomenology of being a john." *Deviant Behavior* 4, no. 1 (1982): 89–116. doi: 10.1080/01639625.1982.9967604.

Hoy.com.ec. 2009. "Doll House, prostíbulo que nunca cierra." Noticias Ecuador. Last modified January 23, 2009. http://www.hoy.com.ec/noticias-ecuador/doll-house-prostibulo-que-nunca-cierra-330345.html.

Huysamen, Monique and Floretta Boonzaier. 2014. "Men's Constructions of Masculinity and Male Sexuality through Talk of Buying Sex." *Culture, Health & Sexuality* 17 (2014): 1–14. doi: 10.1080/13691058.2014.963679.

"Manuela". n.d. "Cómo es vivir en un prostíbulo." *Soho Ecuador*. Accessed February/March 2009. http://www.soho.co/historias/articulo/prostibulos-ser-prostituta-y-vivir-en-un-prostibulo-soho-le-cuenta/9950.

Mirandé, Alfredo. 1997. *Hombres y Machos: Masculinity and Latino Culture*. Boulder: Westview Press.

Nagel, Joane. 2003. *Race, Ethnicity, and Sexuality: Intimate Intersections, Forbidden Frontiers*. New York: Oxford University Press.

Pilar Troya, María. 2001. "No soy machista pero. . .Masculinidades en profesionales de clase media de la ciudad de Quito." In *Masculinidades en Ecuador*, edited by X. Andrade and Gioconda Herrera, 67–97. Quito: FLACSO, Sede Ecuador.

Pitts, Marian K., Anthony M. A. Smith, Jeffrey Grierson, Mary O'Brien, and Sebastian Misson. 2004. "Who Pays for Sex and Why? An Analysis of Social and Motivational Factors Associated with Male Clients of Sex Workers." *Archives of Sexual Behavior* 33, no. 4 (2004): 353–358. doi: 10.1023/B:ASEB.0000028888.48796.4f.

Rogers, Mark. 2003. "Spectacular Bodies: Folklorization and the Politics of Identity in Ecuadorean Beauty Pageants." In *Perspectives on Las Américas: A Reader in Culture, History, and Representation*, edited by Matthew C. Gutmann, Félix V. Matos Rodriguez, Lynn Stephen, and Patricia Zavella, 342–362. Malden: Blackwell Publishing.

Sanders, Teela. 2008. *Paying for Pleasure: Men Who Buy Sex*. Devon: Willan Publishing.

Seal, David W., and Anke. A. Ehrhardt. 2003. "Masculinity and Urban Men: Perceived Scripts for Courtship, Romantic, and Sexual Interactions with Women." *Culture, Health & Sexuality* 5, no. 4 (2003): 295–319. doi: 10.1080/136910501171698.

Soguel, Dominique. n.d. "Ecuador Sex Workers Target HIV-AIDS Prevention." *womensenews.org*. Last modified April 10, 2009. http://www.womensenews.org/story/prostitution-and-trafficking/090410/ecuador-sex-workers-target-hiv-aids-prevention.

Valdés, Teresa and José Olavarría. 1998. *Masculinidades y equidad de género en América Latina*. Santiago: FLACSO-Chile.

Viveros Vigoya, Mara. 2003. "Contemporary Latin American Perspectives on Masculinity." In *Changing Men and Masculinities in Latin America*, edited by Matthew C. Guttman, 27–57. Durham: Duke University Press.

Chapter Four

Becoming Endemic

The Zika Virus Epidemic and Gendered Power in Puerto Rico

Adriana M. Garriga-López
and Carlos E. Rodríguez-Díaz

PREAMBLE

The first case of ZIKV infection in Puerto Rico was confirmed on December 30, 2015. Thereafter, alarming numbers of cases of Zika infection among residents of the unincorporated U.S. territory in 2016 led to the mobilization of numerous federal, state, and local community resources. Yet, the management and delivery of those resources was a highly contentious and deeply gendered process that reflected the existing unequal relations of power between the United States and Puerto Rico, and between differently gendered subjects in Puerto Rico. Ultimately, public health authorities expected the virus to become endemic to the population.

This chapter examines how gendered power structured people's experiences in this process. In particular, large numbers of expected cases among pregnant women in Puerto Rico caused great concern due to the potential severe effects of Zika syndrome on developing fetuses. The prompt discovery of Zika's sexual transmission route meant the virus became ensconced within the long-standing scientific debates around sexually-transmitted infection (STI) transmission generated by HIV/AIDS prevention strategies and interventions. It also led to the implementation of multiple public health strategies meant to ameliorate the potential effects of Zika syndrome and arrive at a greater scientific understanding of the Zika virus and its mechanisms.

We use Charles Rosenberg's (1989) theory of epidemics as a tripartite process of meaning making within social history to look at how the Zika epidemic became a fulcrum for gendered social power in Puerto Rico, and we suggest a fourth "Act" be added to the theory—one in which the story of the epidemic is told by those who wield discursive and institutional power

(Rosenberg 1989). We also discuss how the Zika virus epidemic in the Puerto Rican archipelago points to colonialism, poverty, and gender inequities as the most important barriers to public health on these islands.

FROM THE ZIKA FOREST TO THE ISLANDS OF PUERTO RICO

There are many ways of understanding and addressing an epidemic; from the "germ theory" to combined models that address geological position, climate change, and the social determinants of health. Indisputably, infectious diseases are a predominant cause of morbidity and mortality in many countries around the globe, including Puerto Rico. These diseases have a large social impact that is in some cases related to our limited knowledge of the pathogen and can be exacerbated by the mismanagement of social structures that proscribe risk, provide prevention, and/or properly address their impact. The many negative health outcomes caused by infectious disease epidemics are well documented, including the atrocious results of the poor management of sustained epidemics such as HIV since the 1980s and those of emerging epidemics, such as SARS in the early 2000s, H1N1 in 2009, and MERS since 2012. More recently, we have also experienced the negative health outcomes produced by the epidemics caused by Ebola and Chikungunya.

Zika is a flavavirus transmitted through the bite of the *Aedes sp.* mosquito by sexual contact and blood transfusion. Although the ZIKV outbreak in the Americas started in 2015, ZIKV was first identified in 1947 in the Zika Forest of Uganda. In 1977–1978, it was reported among humans in Pakistan, Malaysia, and Indonesia. In 2007, cases were also reported in Micronesia. More recently, infection was reported in French Polynesia in 2013 and Brazil in 2014. ZIKV infection has been associated with microcephaly and other neurological fetal problems, later named "Zika syndrome." Similarly, several cases of Guillain-Barré syndrome were associated with ZIKV infection. Some studies have shown that ZIKV can also produce negative neurological effects in adults (da Silva et al. 2017).

The first case of the Zika virus in Puerto Rico was confirmed in December of 2015. This stage of the outbreak between the end of 2015 and the first half of 2016 corresponds to the *progressive revelation* phase in Rosenberg's theory of epidemics, during which the growing number of cases leads to the undeniable conclusion that an epidemic is actually taking place (Rosenberg, 1989).

From 2016 to 2017, there were 40,570 confirmed cases of ZIKV in Puerto Rico. Fully 4,035 of these confirmed cases were reported among pregnant women. These case numbers are reliable based on the surveillance system established by the government to document and monitor Zika infections in Puerto Rico. According to the Puerto Rico Department of Health, Zika virus (ZIKV) infection represents one of the most important health problems on the islands since 2016. Nonetheless, there are two main factors that limit our confidence in these reports. First, Zika was an emergent epidemic and, as such, limited knowledge and resources were available to conduct proper health promotion strategies, provide reliable diagnostic tests, or monitor the progression of the epidemic. Second, based on the publicly available data at the Puerto Rico Department of Health, no new cases of Zika were documented in the established surveillance system after the impact of hurricanes Irma and Maria in 2017. In effect, the state simply stopped counting cases after the 2017 hurricane season. Leading local researchers and clinicians have denounced this situation in the media, but to date with no effect (Murphy 2018). We would also like to register our concern that surveillance of Zika virus cases has been abandoned in Puerto Rico since September 2017 and call for the proper oversight and management of this serious health and environmental issue by local public health authorities.

Hurricane Maria and its aftermath laid bare the social inequities that affect Puerto Ricans in regards to health care. In particular, the crisis precipitated by the 2017 hurricane season laid bare how women, poor families, the elderly, people with disabilities, and others are at disproportionate risk for ZIKV and other kinds of communicable diseases, and it exacerbated those vulnerabilities. Thousands of people (including many health professionals) fled the island during the following weeks and months. Many left under duress as a result of health conditions requiring care that was unavailable in Puerto Rico at the time. The health-care system has not yet fully recovered and continues to be under the threat of increased austerity policies due to the ongoing fiscal crisis.

GENDERED CHARACTERISTICS OF THE ZIKA VIRUS IN PUERTO RICO

Zika infection is often asymptomatic. Like other infections that share this characteristic, a significant portion of those infected may not seek medical care. However, asymptomatic carriers can still transmit the infection if no prevention measures are in place. Sexual transmission routes for the Zika virus were confirmed, not before, but during the early months of the Puerto Rican epidemic. This situation of attempting to control risk in a context of fundamental uncertainty corresponds to the second phase in Rosenberg's theorization of epidemics, that of *managing randomness*, which involves "the creation of a framework" for understanding the disease (Rosenberg, 1989).

As scientific and public health knowledge of the virus grew during the epidemic, diagnostic tests were made available, consequences of the infection were better understood, and prevention strategies were implemented. We see this as an example of the third and most complicated phase of epidemics as theorized by Rosenberg, during which a *public response is negotiated,* generating pressure for "decisive and visible community response" (Rosenberg, 1989).

Due to the significant impact of Zika infection in fetuses with neurological and developmental problems, a disproportionate amount of efforts involved women of childbearing age in seeking to prevent the infection or establish care if infected while pregnant. Consistently, more resources were allocated to educate women about how to prevent Zika infection. While education about this emerging pathogen was important for both clinicians and patients, responsibility for vector control was put on people rather than public health institutions, and sexual and reproductive practices became the dominant site for intervention.

As part of the health education campaigns implemented to engage women in Zika management, prevention messages reproduced conservative heteronormative gender norms by assuming that women were responsible for: (1) preventing the propagation of mosquitoes in their households; (2) getting tested if they perceived themselves to be at risk or to have been exposed to the virus; and (3) engaging in preventive sexual practices such as consistent condom use and procuring the use of birth control methods. In addition, abortion as a viable medical alternative for pregnant women with Zika-related complications was seldom discussed or mentioned, despite its legality and availability in Puerto Rico. This situation was protested by feminists and community activists in both public fora and professional conferences, yet these protests had no effect on public health messaging.

PUBLIC HEALTH AND INCREASING WOMEN'S VULNERABILITY

Zika virus infection control efforts were focused on women of childbearing age, especially young women and high school girls. Consequently, more women than men were tested for Zika infection. This may explain the disproportionate amount of confirmed infections among women when compared to men. Similarly, due to the implementation of specific programs targeted to women, such as ZCAN—which favored establishing a network of healthcare providers and clinics to facilitate access to free birth control to women between the ages of 18 and 49 years—more reproductive health services were briefly available to women in Puerto Rico. However, these were temporary in nature, such that the impact of the increased availability of birth control was very limited in scope.

These strategies clearly placed a disproportionate burden on women for controlling Zika infection. While having access to diagnostic tests is essential in the identification and control of pathogens in an epidemic, it's also necessary to involve all the parties at risk. Targeting women in the Puerto Rican Zika prevention campaign perpetuated a lack of balance in assigning responsibilities, especially given that vector control should be a combined effort between households and local public health authorities. These strategies should also be considered in context for Puerto Rico, where high poverty levels impede investing in most of the vector control strategies suggested by public health authorities. Given the economic and fiscal crisis that Puerto Rico has been in since 2006, Zika prevention efforts overly relied on the mobilization of personal resources, thus making them less effective due to their unsystematic distribution and segmentation by socioeconomic class.

Similarly, sexual and reproductive practices are often planned or negotiated with sexual or domestic partners. Targeting women in these efforts was further damaging considering that women, when compared to men, experience more scarcity while in poverty. Likewise, school-based sexual education is practically nonexistent in Puerto Rico due to a long-standing lack of systematic curricula and culturally relevant materials. Therefore, public knowledge about sexual health, as well as the skills needed to make informed reproductive decisions lacks fundamental support. This includes a very limited approach to education about sexuality and gender that fails to challenge traditional and institutionalized power imbalances between men and women.

In addition, the focus on testing among women had the effect of reinforcing the idea that women are responsible for managing the sexual health of their partners. We know that in general women access health care and reproductive care more regularly than men (Carter et al. 2011). Studies about HIV testing have shown that in some cases men will hold off on getting tested in favor of letting their female partners test for HIV and other sexually transmitted infections, thus establishing an unmitigated risk by not testing one of the members of a sexual pair (given that couples can be serodiscordant) and further enforcing women's bodily and affective labor as the precondition for male sexual and mental health (DiCarlo et al. 2014). The over-reliance on testing women for the Zika virus in Puerto Rico further entrenched these already common dynamics with regards to testing for sexually transmitted infections.

By focusing especially on young women's sexual and reproductive choices, the government response to Zika in Puerto Rico also reproduced social norms that portray women as sexually irresponsible, both out of control and in need of state control, therefore rendering young, and especially poor young women and femmes (female-presenting persons, trans women, and non-biological females) vulnerable to sexist power dynamics and a loss of autonomy over their own bodily integrity (Briggs, 2003). In addition, by eliding abortion as an alternative for pregnant women carrying fetuses displaying signs of Zika syndrome, these silences and assumptions also obscured one possible way of avoiding the potentially harrowing and life-long consequences of unintended pregnancies for both women and children.

The health inequities experienced by women due to gender-based discrimination have been previously documented (Baker and Shand, 2017; Vlassof, 2007). While intended to protect health and reduce risks, many public health interventions have also placed the responsibility of using birth control methods mostly on women of reproductive age. In fact, the development of birth control methods is highly biased to women's use of medications (hormones) or medical devices (IUD). In general, the strategies mobilized in order to reduce and impede the enjoyment of reproductive rights are politically influenced. Prominent researchers and activists have called for the development of vaccines and other new technologies that could help mitigate the effects of the Zika virus on the population and on women's reproductive health (Zorrilla et al. 2017).

However, a study conducted in Puerto Rico in the midst of the 2016–2017 outbreak of Zika (Zorrilla et al. 2017) evidenced how sociopolitical and historical factors continue to affect women's decisions about their own bodies. After collecting survey data from 400 men and women, a quarter of the sample (25.9 percent), mainly women (74.3 percent), reported disagreeing with women having access to legal and safe abortion in case of ZIKV infection during pregnancy. Further, 62.9 percent of people who disagreed with access to legal and safe abortions did agree that women should prevent becoming pregnant due to the risk of ZIKV infection. When compared to other religious groups, self-identified Christian participants disagreed more often with women having access to legal and safe abortions in case of being infected with ZIKV during pregnancy. Even though abortions have been legal in Puerto Rico for over forty years, there is still a significant percentage of participants who disagree with women having access to safe abortion. Further, general opinion reported by participants was that women are responsible for preventing pregnancy and for reducing the risk of congenital anomalies.

Focused on vector control, women of reproductive age, and children with birth defects, government responses to ZIKV in Puerto Rico brought two important reproductive rights issues to the fore: first, access to pregnancy termination services, and second, access to and availability of contraceptives. The World Health Organization (WHO) and the United Nations suggested an urgent review of laws and policies to guarantee women's reproductive rights. Despite these recommendations, women in Puerto Rico affected by or at risk of contracting ZIKV continue to experience barriers to accessing their guaranteed rights.

COLONIALISM AS THE ULTIMATE SOCIAL DETERMINANT OF HEALTH

The over 40,000 confirmed cases of Zika infection were reported by a surveillance system operated in Puerto Rico and staffed by the Puerto Rico Department of Health, but its oversight was managed by designated personnel from the Centers for Disease Control and Prevention (CDC). All Zika-related surveillance, diagnostic, treatment, and prevention operations in Puerto Rico were carried out by local personnel under direct management from the CDC in Atlanta, Georgia.

A significant portion of the public health workforce mobilized from the continental United States to the islands to execute CDC mandates had limited knowledge of the country and were appointed for relatively short periods of time as established by CDC deployment policies. These public health professionals spent most of their time "getting to know the island," which included a range of activities from understanding Puerto Rico's politics and geography, to establishing or in some cases re-establishing workgroups, taskforces, and other forms of collaborations with the Puerto Rico Department of Health, local communities, and other organizations including academia and municipal governments.

This experience of operating logistics under procedures developed elsewhere during an emergent epidemic is a clear example of the hurdles experienced in Puerto Rico for the development of proper public health services. While the CDC has the expertise in establishing and monitoring fundamental public health services, the local knowledge and experience needed do not always reside and do not always resonate with CDC leadership or personnel. The CDC serves not only U.S. states and territories, but also globally. Nonetheless, there is limited evidence of the investments dedicated to developing culturally appropriate public health strategies for use in contexts outside the continental United States.

Nearly 50 percent of the population in Puerto Rico lives under the federal poverty level. Women, who are frequently the only source of income for their families and are often underpaid when compared to men, are disproportionally affected by poverty and austerity measures. Poverty is associated with an inability to access adequate health care, including contraceptive methods. As of June 2018, more than 56 percent of children in Puerto Rico live below the economic poverty line, with 84 percent living in high poverty areas (Annie E. Casey Foundation 2018). The enactment of austerity measures is actively increasing the economic gaps, limiting resources available to local governments, and increasing the cost of living in Puerto Rico—including health-care services.

The socioeconomic realities are indissolubly linked to the policies adopted by the Fiscal Control Board established by the PROMESA legislation passed under the Obama administration in 2016. This act of Congress created an undemocratic scenario where the people of Puerto Rico are without democratic representation in their own government and are beholden to pay the costs of financial decisions made by wealthy investors and corrupt government agents. Health outcomes are directly tied to these conditions, as people continue to be left out of the health-care system and the possibility of universal health-care coverage dissipates like so many dreams up in smoke. This impossibility is even more injurious as Puerto Ricans first called health a right and not a privilege during the constitutional convention of 1950–1952, only to have the clause removed from the Puerto Rican Constitution by the U.S. Congress, which required its removal in order to approve the organic act established by the document (Rodríguez-Díaz et al. 2017).

CONCLUSION

In closing, we would like to offer a fourth phase (or "Act") to be added to Rosenberg's theorization of epidemics. This would be the phase of resolution, the establishing of the narrative, or the *telling the story of what happened.* All epidemics eventually wane, though the mechanisms of their dissolution are not always understood. There is often great debate between scientists and clinicians about how exactly successes were won against a particular disease, and there is often contentious debate about the significance or meaning of the experiences associated with the epidemic, among both patients and their communities, and among doctors and scientists alike. The outcome of those debates often shape how societies respond to the next epidemic threat to emerge. Therefore, the *telling the story of what happened* is a crucial component of the historical arc of epidemics and should be considered the final phase in their analysis.

In part but not solely because of the effects of Hurricane Maria, the story of the Zika virus in Puerto Rico is incomplete. Not only are there major gaps in the data, but we still don't have a sense of resolution, nor of an end to the epidemic. Even though it may be ongoing, it has simply receded into the background given the larger and devastating crises that have emerged over the last couple of years on the islands. Researchers, activists, and clinicians have sounded the alarm, but due to the hierarchical structure of medical power in terms of public health issues and the relatively low position of Puerto Rican researchers and clinicians in the medical hierarchy, Puerto Rican public health is very low as a political, social, and economic priority, perhaps its lowest since the islands became a territory of the United States in 1898.

Even if the Zika virus has abated in Puerto Rico, there is currently no evidence to show that is has. Indeed, the mosquito that transmits the virus is endemic to the Caribbean, so even if the number of active cases has declined, the virus is now part of the natural reservoir, leading to the possibility of new infections and renewed spread of the disease at any time.

Differently positioned actors within various structures of gendered power, including governmental, grassroots, and public health organizations (among others) influenced the discourse on the Zika virus in Puerto Rico in unequal, yet mutually implicated ways. The outcomes of their discursive battles and negotiations determined what actions were taken to ameliorate the epidemic. In the end, those with institutional and social power may have the last word on how the story is told, but it is our responsibility as social scientists to point out what the official narratives obscure and withhold.

This outbreak of the Zika virus and the stories that we tell about its significance highlight the necessity of understanding and comprehensively addressing the sociopolitical determinants of health that produce and reproduce health inequalities. Our analysis shows these were critical determinants in the spread and management of the Zika virus in Puerto Rico. Finally, these conditions make tangible the deep connections between Puerto Rico as a U.S. colony and neocolonial dynamics in the Caribbean and South America where the virus also caused great social alarm and personal concern but led to little public accountability.

WORKS CITED

Annie E. Casey Foundation. "2018 Kids Count Data Book: State Trends in Child Well-Being," 2018.

Baker, Peter and Tim Shand. "Men's health: time for a new approach to policy and practice?" *Journal of Global Health* 7 no. 1 (2017): 010306.

Briggs, Laura. *Reproducing Empire: Race, Sex, Science, and U.S. Imperialism in Puerto Rico*. University of California Press, 2003.

Carter, Marion W., Joan Marie Kraft, Kendra Hatfield-Timajchy, Linda Hock-Long, and Matthew Hogben. "STD Testing Behaviors Among Black and Puerto Rican

Young Adults," *Perspectives on Sexual and Reproductive Health 43* no. 4 (2011): 238–246.

da Silva, Ivan Rocha Ferreira, Jennifer A. Frontera, Ana Maria Bispo de Filppis, Osvaldo Jose Moreira do Nascimento, and the RIO-GBS-DIKV Research Group. "Neurologic Complications Associated with the Zika Virus in Brazilian Adults," *JAMA Neurology 74* no. 10 (2017): 1190–1198.

DiCarlo, Abby, Joanne E. Mantell, Robert H. Remien, Allison Zerbe, Danielle Morris, Blanche Pitt, Elaine J. Abrams, and Wafaa El-Sadr. "'Men usually say that HIV testing is for women': Gender dynamics & perceptions of HIV testing in Lesotho," *Culture, Health & Sexuality 16* no. (2014): 867–882.

Murphy, Beth. "What's the truth about Zika virus in post-hurricane Puerto Rico?," PBS Newshour, Nov. 14, 2018. https://www.pbs.org/newshour/show/whats-the-truth-about-zika-virus-in-post-hurricane-puerto-rico

Rodríguez-Díaz, Carlos, Adriana Garriga-López, Souhail M. Malavé-Rivera, and Ricardo L. Vargas-Molina. "Zika virus epidemic in Puerto Rico: Health justice too long delayed," *International Journal of Infectious Diseases 65* (2017): 144–147.

Rosenberg, Charles E, "What is an Epidemic? AIDS in Historical Perspective," *Daedalus 118* no. (1989): 1–17.

Vlassof, Carol. "Gender Differences in Determinants and Consequences of Health and Illness." *Journal of Health, Population and Nutrition 25* no. 1 (2007): 47–61.

Zorrilla, Carmen D., Inés García García, Lourdes García Fragoso, and Alberto de la Vega. "Zika Virus Infection in Pregnancy: Maternal, Fetal, and Neonatal Considerations," *Journal of Infectious Diseases 216* no. 10 (2017): S891–S896.

Chapter Five

Gender and Conceptualizing Concern for Sickle Cell Disease in Guadeloupe

Shan-Estelle Brown

Around World Sickle Cell Day, June 19, I attended a dinner event celebrating families affected by sickle cell disease in Guadeloupe. Guadeloupe, the overseas region of France, has at least two private organizations formed to provide families with sickle cell disease with information and a social network. This event was big. Held in a warehouse, it was the longest dinner I have ever attended, probably so that people would feel like they had received their money's worth for the admission ticket. There were a series of events including spoken word poetry, a few bands, a silent auction, a dance party with a DJ, and there was even a magician for the children. Unfortunately, the catered food became dry while waiting for more guests to arrive. The event was not well attended. By the end of the night, around 1:00 a.m., the majority of the seats at each table were still not filled. I also noticed that the majority of the organizers and attendees were women. Where was everyone? Where were the men? Although parents contribute 50 percent of their DNA to offspring, the burden of caring for a child with sickle cell disease is not shared equally. In an interview with a social worker that treats sickle cell patients, I learned that people in Guadeloupe are concerned about being seen and labeled as "the parent with the sick kid." For these parents, the label is a constant reminder that their child is sick and possibly dying, and this can be a source of shame. In this chapter I argue that genetic risk and the potential consequences of sickle cell disease are disproportionately placed on women as bearers of children and as "pillars of society" both in the public sphere and within their families, which places the responsibility for the cultural value of looking infallible in society on both men and women.

BACKGROUND

Guadeloupe has a high prevalence of sickle cell disease, a genetic disease of malformed red blood cells that predominantly affects people of African and Mediterranean descent. In Guadeloupe, one in eight citizens is a carrier for sickle cell disease and one in 260 babies born each year in Guadeloupe has sickle cell disease (Tarer et al. 2006). My two longest trips to Guadeloupe were bookended by an economic strike in 2009 that interrupted the majority of activities occurring in the archipelago. These political and economic tensions between "hexagonal France" and a resistant *Département* continued to color conversations in my interviews. For example, one respondent referred to Guadeloupe as "a country of strikes" (Interview 12) in the sense that everyone has to deal with the inconvenience associated with whatever others are striking against. The stereotype of Guadeloupe is that it is an island paradise where people live by the Creole motto "*pa ni pwoblem*" (no problems) and yet some people experience significant stress.

THE BASICS OF SICKLE CELL DISEASE

Sickle cell disease (SCD) is an autosomal recessive genetic disease, meaning that someone can be a heterozygous carrier for the disease but have no symptoms. If two people are genetic carriers and have children together, each potential child has a 25 percent chance of having this congenital disease, a 50 percent chance of being a carrier, and a 25 percent chance of having normal genes (Wille et al. 2004). For health education, outreach efforts are complicated due to the nature of sickle cell disease being genetic and that in areas where newborn screenings are longstanding and well-conducted, genetic knowledge about carrier status might be known, but still requires knowledge of a partner's status. The concept of genetic risk is difficult for lay people to understand for three reasons. The first is because it involves the potentiality of having a child with a genetic disease. Second, in addition to possibly shaky understandings of genetics, people are also removed from the impact of the disease in the sense that they are not directly afflicted—their children are. Third, sickle cell disease is rare enough that either most people are unaware of it, even if locally there is a significant prevalence of the disease. Even most medical professionals in the United States are unaware of how to treat sickle cell disease. In medical school, sickle cell disease is presented as an abstraction, a test case for understanding genetics, which is divorced from actual lived experiences.

Inside the body of a person with sickle cell disease, red blood cells that would normally be spongy, soft, and round collapse into a sickle shape, which is problematic for moving through tiny capillaries. These misshaped red blood cells tend to create blockages in blood vessels, particularly in the extremities, which cause intense pain episodes called crises. These crises appear as early as at birth and continue through the lifespan. This pain takes a toll on organs and it is usually organ failure that causes premature death for people with sickle cell disease. For people who have known someone with sickle cell disease, they know that the lived experience could be painful and tragically short.

Outside the body, this pain is racialized in interpretation, and sickle cell disease is widely considered "a black disease." Attitudes toward sickle cell disease and black and brown bodies in pain have been increasingly witnessed and documented since the late 1990s. Historian Keith Wailoo's book *Dying in the City of the Blues* (2001) traced the history of sickle cell disease both before and after it was "discovered" by Western medicine; the book also weaves together illness experiences of African Americans with their relationship to the predominantly white medical establishment, holding up a mirror to American society to show how race and health are intertwined. The majority of the research on sickle cell disease still comes from the United States, a nation with a long and diligent history of systemic racism embedded in its medical institutions (Feagin and Bennefield 2014). Because of existing structural discrimination against African Americans, sickle cell disease and its pain have traditionally been understudied and are therefore not well understood. There is a history of medical professionals undertreating sickle cell pain, applying unconscious bias that African Americans can withstand more pain, and assuming patients are people with drug problems looking for pain medication (Weisberg et al. 2013, Ballas, Gupta, and Adams-Graves 2012, Haywood Jr et al. 2010, Zempsky 2009).

SOCIAL SCIENCE ON SICKLE CELL DISEASE

Social science research worldwide, and rightfully so, has focused on assessing the lived experiences of people with sickle cell disease in the hope of improving health outcomes, fostering better relationships with sickle cell patients and their medical providers, and reducing wait times for hospital and emergency room visits for people experiencing crises. Other issues of sickle cell disease address interpretations of ancestry and territory (Carter and Dyson 2011), how race and attitudes toward SCD are intertwined in hospital settings (Bediako and Haywood Jr 2009, Bediako and Moffitt 2011), how to provide care for children with sickle cell disease (Ahmad and Atkin 1996), disclosing sickle cell disease to others (Dyson et al. 2010), newborn screening programs (Ducrocq et al. 2001, Frampton 1990, Galacteros 1996, Grossman et al. 1985), assessing attitudes toward genetic screening and prenatal diagnosis (Atkin et al. 2008, Ahmed, Green, and Hewison 2006), strategies for providing genetic screening tests to people with genetic risk (Berghs, Dyson, and Atkin 2015), and assessing public awareness of hemoglobinopathies (Al Arrayed and Al Hajeri 2010, Savas et al. 2010). This research has resulted in some changes to hospital settings, such as the creation of dedicated clinics for sickle cell patients, and increases in clinical trial research to identify better treatments such as the medication hydroxyurea (Wong et al. 2014, Segal and Johns Hopkins University Evidence-based Practice Center 2008) and advancements in bone marrow transplants, which have shown some promise in a potential cure. These are optimistic updates in sickle cell disease.

Although this recent research focus has been beneficial, families experiencing sickle cell disease have still been waiting a long time for the biomedical community to pay attention to their needs (Brown, Weisberg, and Sledge 2015). Lay caregivers of sickle cell patients and the patients themselves have had to be the most lionhearted defenders, informed patient advocates, educators of medical professionals, and comfort during terrible crises. Sickle cell disease, having a lower priority in the medical world than other diseases, has shaped my own research trajectory; after finishing my doctorate, I began studying HIV because of more available funding opportunities to better understand gaps in the HIV continuum of care, and the stages of medical care that a person living with HIV moves through from diagnosis to getting into care and receiving antiretroviral medications with the goal of reaching viral suppression. The spread of HIV represents a clarion call for more testing and treatment in ways that rarer diseases like sickle cell disease have never received. Today, a significant growth area in sickle cell disease research is happening in the lab, not in communities, in the form of gene therapy using stem cells (Talano and Cairo 2015) and gene editing to correct the genetic mutation that causes sickle cell disease (Bourzac 2017). Although these studies are long overdue for families waiting for a cure for sickle cell disease, the scientific placement of SCD research in laboratories means that there is less focus to investigate people-centered issues of SCD, such as inequality in medical care, nor does it make sense to research barriers and facilitators to adherence for treatments that do not yet exist for people affected by the disease.

In anthropology, debates continue about how anthropologists should discuss race and racism (Lieberman and Kirk 2004), with one study showing that even anthropology textbooks seem to be moving away from discussions of race and racism (Shanklin 2000). There are also speculations about how the "new genetics" (the inclusion and involvement of genetic information into multiple facets of society) will affect perceptions of genetic risk and race-based interpretations of heredity, particularly an emphasis on avoiding risk with respect to reproductive genetics (Ettorre 2002). There are also significant differences between lay and professional interpretations of genetics, as Rayna Rapp argues (Rapp 1998, 1997).

Apart from research on the prevalence of the sickle cell gene by biological anthropologists dating to the 1950s, the social effects of sickle cell disease have specifically been studied by a handful of recent medical anthropologists, sometimes in collaboration with medical professionals or in the form of ethnographic research conducted in biomedical settings such as Paula Tanabe's research in emergency departments (Brennan-Cook et al. 2018, Glassberg, Tanabe, Richardson, et al. 2013, Glassberg, Tanabe, Chow, et al. 2013, Haywood Jr et al. 2013, Tanabe et al. 2010). Melbourne Tapper's book *In the Blood: Sickle Cell Anemia and the Politics of Race* (1999) explains how sickle cell disease was used to promote white supremacy and racial purity, especially since some populations are targeted for sickle cell screening based on phenotype. Carolyn Moxley Rouse studied SCD in hospital settings in the United States for the ethnography *Uncertain Suffering* (2009) which examines inequality among pediatric black American sickle cell disease patients. Rouse argues that racism, attitudes about pain and suffering, and patients' use of health care designed for poor people are contributors to disparities in care. In the twentieth century, medical advancements have significantly lengthened the lifespan of people with sickle cell disease. The most recent statistics on life expectancy are age forty-two years for men and forty-eight years for women (Lanzkron, Carroll, and Haywood 2013), which is double what physicians traumatically told adult sickle cell patients as children: that they would not live to see adulthood (Brown, Weisberg, and Sledge 2015), and yet today these patients are parents to teenagers.

The research article "You Just Have to Live with It": Coping With Sickle Cell Disease in Jamaica" (Anderson and Asnani 2013) was the first qualitative study on Jamaicans' experiences with SCD and identified themes of loss that SCD inflicted on people and attempts to regain control over SCD by forgetting about it. Medical providers frequently put their own medical authority above the lived experiences of their patients by questioning patients' use of medical resources and requests for pain medication, which made concerns of SCD patients delegitimized and invisible, as Ciribassi and Patil (2016) identified in interviews. The theme of delegitimization also appears in Monica Mann's (2010) biomedical and ethnomedical interpretations of a Togolese immigrant in New York City who has a sickle cell crisis in a public subway and experiences one misunderstanding after another as he suffers from real pain. Duana Fullwiley's research in Senegal began with a question of what genetic screening for Islamic Senegalese families would look like. She identifies discriminate biopower in that larger ministries of health overlook SCD to focus on health priorities deemed more important; she also presents the cultural value of having children and tensions between traditional biomedical techniques and modern techniques of genetic testing, as well as gauging interest in even knowing genetic testing results (Fullwiley 2004, 2010, 2012).

THEORETICAL APPROACH AND METHODS

My research study is grounded in the anthropological debates presented here and uses the concepts presented in Carter and Dyson's (2011) article "Territory, Ancestry and Descent: The Politics of Sickle Cell Disease." In it, the authors show how the notions of race, ethnicity, and ancestry are all social constructions that genetic testing claims to connect "in a more 'authentic' and 'revealing' way," using sickle cell disease as the exemplar (2011: 967). Here, I also use sickle cell disease to argue that local interpretations of this disease cannot be understood without knowledge of the history behind how Guadeloupe came to be, socially, culturally, and politically. Sickle cell disease, therefore, is directly related to the movements of peoples to Guadeloupe, attachment to the land, and delineations between what makes someone *from* Guadeloupe. Through these processes, gender relations between men and women become apparent.

Using a framework of critical medical anthropology, I investigate how a disease like sickle cell disease is situated in social contexts in Guadeloupe. Diseases and medical procedures represent intersections of power, class, race, gender, and culture. Gender affects how people in Guadeloupe see (1) who gets sick, (2) whose responsibility it is to stay well, (3) who should discuss illness, (4) who can discuss his or her own illnesses and with whom, and (5) who seeks health care. Through one-on-one interviews, I also asked about relationships between Guadeloupean men and women, and how sickle cell disease reinforces and conflicts with these relationships. Specifically, I used Handwerker's (2002) explanation of culture in that each individual is multicultural and shares some thoughts, life experiences, emotions, and behaviors with other individuals, and that the shared experiences give rise to culture. I also used cultural consensus theory to identify cultural models of sickle cell disease and a critical medical anthropology approach to account for political and economic factors that might explain possible health inequities in knowledge, attitudes, and behaviors about this disease. Finally, I used Kleinman's Explanatory Model of Illness (Helman 2000) as a supplement to this project's theoretical framework, since it is important to understand how individuals perceive sickle cell disease and related procedures such as carrier screening.

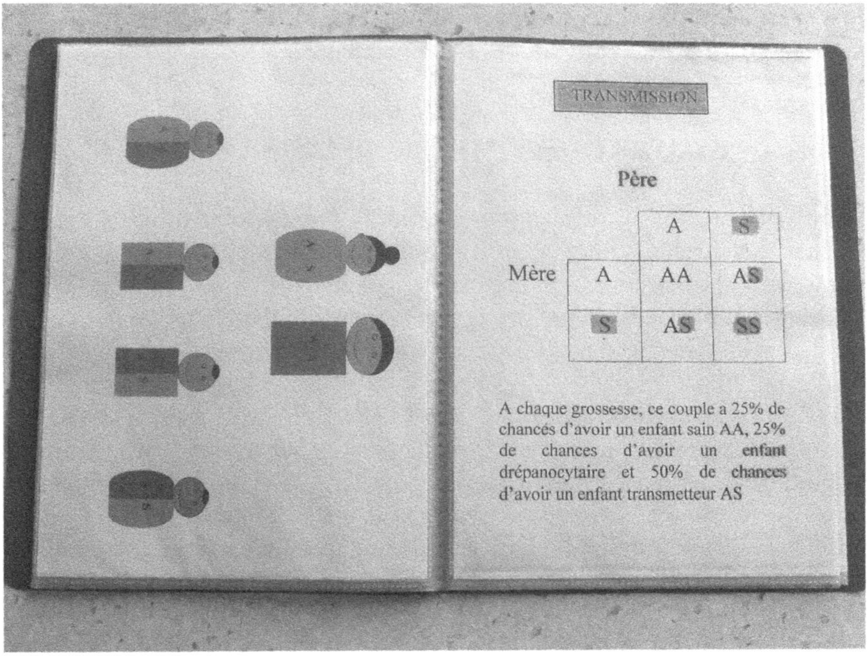

Figure 5.1.
Image taken by author. Figure translation: "At each pregnancy, this couple has a 25% chance of having a healthy child, a 25% chance of having a child with sickle cell anemia, and a 50% chance of having a child who is an asymptomatic sickle cell anemia carrier."

This paper presents interview findings from a larger mixed-methods study conducted primarily in 2010 with a follow-up field visit in 2013. I was based at the sickle cell clinic Unité Transversale de La Drépanocytose at Centre Hospitalier Universitaire (CHU) in the capital Pointe à Pitre. The clinic tests and educates adults and cares for individuals with sickle cell disease. For example, figure 5.1 is educational material from the clinic and is used to educate parents about the importance of getting tested for sickle cell disease prior to becoming pregnant.

In all, 32 semi-structured interviews were conducted in different locations in Guadeloupe, some with a trained research assistant who was a medical student. I hired two transcriptionists to transcribe all interviews conducted in the field from the audio recorder into text. The research assistant and I identified subtleties in the informants' responses. I coded the interviews using content analysis after my return to the United States. I also coded the field notes as described by Emerson, Fretz, and Shaw (1995). The interviews and field notes were coded and analyzed with the computer program ATLAS.ti® to find meaningful similarities in how respondents perceived issues related to sickle cell disease and carrier testing. This project was funded by the National Science Foundation's Doctoral

Dissertation Improvement Grant and was approved by the Institutional Review Board of the University of Connecticut.

GUADELOUPE, THE "SECRET" PARADISE

To only the most well-traveled tourists, Guadeloupe is known for its tropical beaches, local rums, "fiery" Creole cuisine (Ashenburg 1990), sailing competitions, and zouk music. Otherwise, Guadeloupe is a secret. The tagline for a tourism piece about Guadeloupe for readers in the United States called Guadeloupe, "islands that the French have been keeping for themselves" (Wallraff 2002).

On some maps of Guadeloupe, the small "Fr" or all-caps "FRANCE" after Guadeloupe's name speaks volumes about its history. Guadeloupe's economic and political situation as a *Département* is described in an international real estate magazine (2015) as "subsidized by France;" I am confident that this phrase would offend local people in Guadeloupe because the phrase reinforces the archipelago's dependence on France while all but disavowing its history of slavery and colonialism in the entire Caribbean region. In fact, Guadeloupe has undergone serious introspection and political, institutional, and ongoing cultural change during a significant period of decolonization (Bangou 2001, 1987, 1988) since its change in status from territory to *Département*. Yet, one travel writer described Guadeloupe as a prize not only won, but kept:

> France once traded hulking Canada for the butterfly-shaped Caribbean island of Guadeloupe, and—without wishing to ruffle any flannels among the lumberjacks—in the bleak midwinter, at least, it's easy to see why it might have struck that bargain. Actually a cluster of small islands, Guadeloupe has all the classic elements of a tropical paradise: white, pink and black sand beaches; tropical jungles protected in national parks that don't subsidize logging; towering waterfalls with delightful swimming holes at their bases; scuba and snorkeling galore; even a smoldering volcano and a couple of reasonably hot discos. Add to that authentic Creole culture, French patisseries, local sugar that is distilled into local rum, local coffee, local chocolate and—well, let's just say that by 1763 beaver hats weren't selling as briskly in Paris as they had, and the deal with the British for Canada was quietly done. (Schneider 2006)

Guadeloupe is much less known by tourists from English-speaking countries, and there are some French citizens who have never traveled to Guadeloupe, yet most French Antillean people have lived in France for some period of time. Because of recent airline campaigns that have started flights or added flights to Guadeloupe in the last few years, visiting Guadeloupe has become much more easily accessible to tourists looking for a different kind of Caribbean experience that is more French and less touristy than other islands.

LOCAL COLOR: THE COMPLEXITY OF GUADELOUPE

I should first start by explaining that not everyone agrees about who counts as being Guadeloupean, especially since some people may have been born in France but raised in Guadeloupe from childhood, or vice versa; all the participants had some experience living and working in Europe, and the migration patterns between France and Guadeloupe are frequent and based primarily on where jobs are available. Guadeloupean identity is based on race, prioritizing brown skin over white, followed by birthplace. Thus, a white person who was either born in Guadeloupe or lived his entire life in Guadeloupe would often be mistaken for being *zoreil*, a pejorative term for white strangers from France. There is also a skin color hierarchy among brown skin tones with the *chabin* (to describe a woman: *chabine*) at the top: a black person with very light skin tone, blond, frizzy hair, and gray eyes, the result of generations of mixing between Europeans and Africans. For one participant, the idea of being Guadeloupean is really just a byproduct of having been descended from ancestors who were brought there as enslaved people: "The fact that we are Guadeloupean is because we are on this island is all" (Interview 7). This man's response connects to the idea of broader West Indian culture, with the Creole language being the uniting language of people across the Caribbean, regardless of nationality or other languages spoken.

To begin to understand Guadeloupe is to understand that it is a region of France with a racially black (or as one man put it, "bronzed" [Interview 20]) majority that experiences post-colonial tensions with France, especially since it is part of the French state. Residents thought it was especially important for me to understand how Guadeloupe interacts with the rest of France. There is a sentiment that France does not fully fulfill its promises of "liberty, equality, and fraternity" for the people of Guadeloupe, which creates a continuous dialogue about French identity, black French identity, and Antillean identity. One woman, a fashion designer, told me that Guadeloupean youth have embraced their blackness and begun to question France about its obligations in ways that older, more materialistic Guadeloupeans have not: "as I tell them, France brings us equality, fraternity. But what is it? This is only [a] demo. When one is a free people in his head, one day, one sits and asks. We ask for the meanings of these words. And I tell myself that for our young children, not the old ones because they are camped in their cars, in their buildings. They are well nursed, now they are all materialistic, they are confused. They have confused values" (Interview 24). Followed by outward racial appearance, place of birth is important to Guadeloupean identity: "A Guadeloupean is not necessarily someone who was born in Guadeloupe already. Because there are many people who came after, finally in adolescence, even later, who are Guadeloupean. And I think they are well integrated" (Interview 15).

France, not France

Guadeloupean residents are French citizens with the same rights, the same abilities, and the same duties as other French citizens, or as my research assistant said to me, "a true French person." Residents of Guadeloupe have the benefits of having French citizenship, the beauty of the Caribbean, and access to well-organized institutions such as the medical system. In informal conversations where I would introduce my research, people would refer me to the central hospital that has a sickle cell center for screening and care, not yet knowing that I was where I was based. Participants spoke highly of the medical system: "Even if we have no money we get treatment. The only problem is that for specialists we sometimes have to wait a long time" (Interview 3). Participants also stated that most social services worked well, apart from when strikes occurred. Regarding people with disabilities, the Guadeloupean anthropologist I interviewed stated that there are laws to protect people with disabilities, and "people cannot be fired, lose their jobs anyhow. They can check their incapacity to work. So the employers, to my knowledge, have not used this case consistently" (Interview 23). I interviewed a man with sickle cell disease who said that employers would rather not hire someone with disabilities and essentially circumvent the law: "[people who are] disabled, they have difficulty finding a job. It's real in fact. Employers refuse to take disabled people into companies for various reasons. Sometimes, the state forces them to hire disabled people; they prefer to pay taxes for not hiring disabled people. And that's why the state has increased taxes, raised taxes" (Interview 22).

In Guadeloupe there is also a plurality of identities, since people are Guadeloupean and also French: "I still possess Guadeloupe culture. So yes, I'm French, I have a French nationality, I live on the French territory, I have all the rights of a real French from the bottom, but I have a Guadeloupe culture, which is still heritage from here and that others do not have there" (Interview 14). Although Guadeloupe is considered a "black" or "brown" country to Guadeloupeans, there is very little cultural reference to the African continent, as if people have chosen to be Guadeloupean and fight for French equality; ties to Africa seem to be ancestral and grounded in the past rather than present-day African nations. Within Guadeloupe, the complex hierarchy of Guadeloupean society is expressed in a variety of ways, such as comedy (Managan 2012), and the social placement of Haitians as immigrants in the lower rungs. Despite having the fourth-largest Indian community in the Caribbean, having been brought as laborers from southern India, Indians are culturally absent (Bonilla 2015). The hierarchy shifts outside Guadeloupe, however. Despite the assumption of equality, Guadeloupean people were quick to tell me about how the French emphasize differences between themselves and people from the Antilles in a way that maintains French (and therefore, white) dominance over others, and prioritize the French state in Europe, which makes everything else a backwater and backward hinterland. One example of the emphasis on differences came from one respondent: "on the news if there is a robbery, if it is someone from the West Indies, it will be specified in national news. They will say 'a Guadeloupean, a person of Caribbean origin, or of Maghreb origin, or. . . .' If it's someone from France, they will never specify" (Interview 14). She further explained that after a visit to France, she called Guadeloupe a territory: the French "know it is a French territory but as we are far away, they make it a difference by saying , 'Yes, but it's not France.'"

A result of Guadeloupean enculturation is local pride; people I spoke to were proud of being from Guadeloupe. As one woman said, "I admit that I give a lot of importance to the fact that I come from here" (Interview 14). Another participant said in an interview, "you have to be very proud to be born here" (Interview 20). It was sometimes difficult for participants to explain what counts as Guadeloupean culture. One quote that I like is: "Beyond culture, it's the philosophy. It's a rhythm" (Interview 17).

DOMINATION AND WEAKNESS

The historical institution of slavery permeates conversations about power and geopolitics between France and Guadeloupe. There is a common narrative about enslaved peoples in history as powerless to shape their own destinies. Using material remains such as ceramics, archaeologist Myriam Arcangeli (2015) directly confronts this narrative by focusing on the role of enslaved women as valuable cooks who built the framework for the Creole cuisine that so many people enjoy today. As one person in my interviews stated, "We have always been necessarily bathed in stories where we have endured a lot of slavery. And therefore one has a refusal to be too dominated or too much to walk on another person's feet. So no, that's the way most people say, 'That's enough, we're free, we've endured enough. This time we get up, we assume and we refuse'" (Interview 17). For this reason, the economic strikes are particularly entrenched and disruptive.

At the community level, in Guadeloupean culture there is a sense of jealousy between people in the same community, and as people begin to find ways to explain differences in who has advanced socially or financially, magic might factor in the explanation. As explained by a Guadeloupean anthropologist, "magic is the explanation for why bad things happen to people: people who are in social competition in a given neighborhood, seeing that such family is influential in the social ladder, earns more money, children succeed in school, and etc., will be jealous of this family and will cast a spell on it. But in reality, no one has cast a spell on anyone" (Interview 22). Magic, therefore, was the explanation for sickle cell disease before science could explain problems in blood cells: "It was only from the moment that we were able to define precisely what were the origins of sickle cell disease that at that time we were able to give a scientific explanation to the problem that people had encountered before" (Interview 23).

Despite biomedical knowledge about Guadeloupe, it seems that people associated with SCD experience shame and stigma. When I asked the man with sickle cell disease whom I interviewed if he cared if the general public knew he had the disease, he said, "I would not want people to know that. Other than my friends or family but otherwise after that, people get pissed at my fate and then they see it as a weak point" (Interview 22). I believe that since he is male, the desire to look as if he doesn't have weaknesses is also based in gender as well as perceptions of sickle cell disease as debilitating. As an extension of the power difference between individuals, my research assistant explained that Guadeloupeans are constantly on the lookout for what they call *petites dominations* (little dominations). Examples of *petites dominations* are when a person knows someone else's possessions, particularly their brand or quality, and uses that information against them, borrows possessions without returning them, or asks to borrow possessions after he or she has already taken them. Health information is also a possession, and losing control of health information to people who gossip could mean that a minor health issue could be magnified into people thinking a person has AIDS, which is considered one of the worst-case health scenarios. By watching out for gossips and generally, anyone who is curious about someone else's life, one can protect oneself from being dominated (Interview 13).

RELATIONS BETWEEN MEN AND WOMEN IN GUADELOUPE

In her research on the 2009 economic strike in Martinique, Camee Maddox (2015) points out that French feminism is not intersectional and does not examine race, gender, and class. It appears that the 2009 strike put race at the forefront of the economic problems and pushed gender to the rear, even though it is well documented that women have been involved in revolutions in the French Caribbean. Women's gender roles seem to be somewhat rigid and mediated by the assumed level of crime, and so the use of *associations* in Guadeloupe, the equivalent of social clubs or non-profit organizations, provides a safer space for women to congregate, socialize, and lead (Managan 2015). This is possibly the reason for the few numbers of men at the association dinner I attended for World Sickle Cell Day. In her interviews with women in Guadeloupean associations, Kathe Managan (2015) found that they reported that men were able to do many more things in public than they could do.

This research recognizes the social importance of women, particularly mothers, as the *poto mitan*, the pillar of the family unit; this cultural phenomenon was shaped by colonialism and slavery, when male slaves lacked agency over their own lives—at least, this is how participants explained it to me. Thus, the belief in Guadeloupe today is that men and women are equal genetic contributors to their children, but their influence upon their children's lives has different proportions and purposes. Guadeloupean men and women are assumed to be heterosexual. Since sexual reproduction generates children and some children with SCD, one would think that sexuality takes a strong precedence in the study of SCD, but it does not—not in the literature and not in the way SCD is discussed among participants I have directly encountered and interviewed in the United States and in Guadeloupe. Discussions about sickle cell disease occur "post sex"—this is actually problematic, since some people are unaware of sickle cell disease *until* the birth of a child. If anything, the emphasis is on the power of social relationships and the fear of others knowing one's genetic risk or any other issue that could be construed as a frailty by someone else. It is also possible that participants were uncomfortable discussing sexuality with me. For this reason, this chapter focuses on gender and how it is socially constructed, rather than sexuality.

As was explained to me across the interviews, in West Indian society, men and women are not equal. From one interviewee: "The man will always feel superior to the woman here. Well it is the case everywhere on earth, but it is more here anyway that compared to the city for example, it is more pronounced here anyway" (Interview 20). Men and women have different roles. Participants initially hesitated to share stereotypes about men and women in Guadeloupe, which is understandable and polite; however, their responses are similar across the interviews.

From the interviews, Guadeloupean men are bad drivers, chauvinists, slackers, not necessarily very courteous, but generous, who know how to welcome someone when they feel like it (Interview 20). Men are considered strong (Interview 14) and macho "because of the temperature" (Interview 20) as opposed to women who are considered weak: "He almost thinks that the woman, because she is a woman, she is weak" (Interview 14). The interview conversation would then gravitate into sexual matters: "The Guadeloupean man loves to live. He likes to live beyond his means . . . he's a seducer. It's the rooster of the barnyard" (Interview 15). Men are expected to have numerous sexual conquests (Interview 13), and even maintain simultaneous relationships. As one man explained, "Our official wife is our wife. And there are the mistresses next door. These are the men. And there are some women who accept that. Here, for appearances. So they pretend they do not see" (Interview 14). From a different interview, a participant told me that the Guadeloupean man is respectful in that he is not a violent man when his sexual advances are rebuffed: "When a woman is going to say 'no' to him, he will not insist . . . he will insist, but he will not try to violate her" (Interview 15).

Women are often considered gossips, with the alternative being the *poto mitan* in families where women make decisions (Interview 14). From one interview, the respondent told me that Caribbean women are quite independent and have a strong character (Interview 20), which seems in contrast to the stereotype that women are weak. As one participant explained, "even if I see her in relation to the man who thinks she is weak, they have a strong character anyway" (Interview 14). Women are more attentive to their health than men are (Interview 16). The more prevailing view is that the woman is in complete control of the household, and if the man is making a decision, it is because the woman is allowing it to happen: "The man is going to bring back the money and the food but after that it's the woman who runs the house, who runs the expenses, and the children, and all that. Yes, she is in charge of everything. And the West Indian man is lazy as he is so anyway, he does not bother too much" (Interview 20).

Both men and women value children, but for women, the circumstance of pregnancy seems to matter. Women are expected to have few sexual conquests. As one man explained, "If a woman gets married pregnant, we say that it's *because* she's pregnant that she gets married. . . . A woman who gets pregnant when the father is unknown is said to carry 'her burden.' As the father, I can go anywhere, get one or two girls pregnant, but I'm not aware. And then I can ask them to prove that I am their dad, there is no proof" (Interview 14). Motherhood is of special importance:

> Women make the decisions, often the man agrees. When it is not necessarily it creates problems but they are often the engines of family decisions. I'm going to take the expression that comes up all the time, "*se on Guadloupéen, se on poto mitan*" ("they are Guadeloupean, they are the middle pillar"). Finally I find that

> here, the family is very matriarchal. It's really the mother. She does everything. I think that is the case everywhere since it is the role that has always been given to women to take care of children, to make food. But I find that here, she takes care of the other side of her family too: her brothers, her sisters. (Interview 15)

Despite the numerous references to the Guadeloupean woman as a mother, there was also recognition that gender roles have changed significantly over the twentieth century:

> The gender roles used to be more separate and more rigid, and now women are much more active as breadwinners outside the home. It's two generations before us. It is a little less for our parents. Because already at the time of our parents was the time when women began to emancipate, began to work, began to have other activities. This is even less true now. Even if we find a little, but it will be nuanced because the West Indian woman is no longer the housewife who raises children, it is the West Indian woman active. (Interview 14)

The opinion about women's roles having changed over time was reinforced in a separate interview: "Now everyone is working but bringing back the money and are in positions of responsibility, but the central figure is the mother. And the mother has an important role and often it erases the men around. It is mothers who make decisions for the family, if there is a problem it is the mother who settles the problem, the mother has her say and when she speaks, she listens. And the mother influences the father and the father will execute his authority in relation to the opinion of the mother. The mother will make the decision and dad will follow the decision, follow suit and assume his role as father of authority" (Interview 8).

EXPLANATIONS OF SICKLE CELL DISEASE IN GUADELOUPE

Colonial ties and the history of slavery become incorporated into the Guadeloupean explanations about how sickle cell disease came to Guadeloupe. A Guadeloupean male anthropologist I interviewed said, "When we go back to genetics and we see the part that slavers have taken in the miscegenation of the country, after, the combinations. . . . Add to that the arrival of the Indians of India, so that's still other combinations. We do not stop at that moment" (Interview 23). This sentiment is mirrored in another response: "Europeans arrived [in Guadeloupe], they killed all the Arawak that were here, all the Indians and Americans that were here. They came to get us the Africans, they took us back there, they slept with them, it was mixed and then we arrived. So if there were no slaves, I'm sorry, there would have been only whites who would have made whites pay for them. There would have been no slavery. There would have been white employees and there would have been no Guadeloupeans as we know them now. And there might not have been sickle cell disease either" (Interview 20). There are also counter-narratives about slavery becoming the explanation for everything wrong in Guadeloupe. The fashion designer I interviewed explained that, at this point, the problem is internal: "West Indian people have a strength of soul . . . we are a strong people" and "the problem is not in slavery, the problem is with us. We must now look in our values and stop" (Interview 24).

HAVING CHILDREN AS A CARRIER

The individuals whom I interviewed held strong opinions about how carriers of sickle cell disease should proceed with this knowledge, as far as having children was concerned, but there was not a consensus about whether or not parents were to blame for their children being sick with SCD. In fact, participants seemed to resist assigning blame. For one participant, parents of a child with SCD should not be blamed: "I would not say it's his fault but . . . at the same time a child, his parents gave him life so it's beautiful, but afterwards, in a way the child is a burden, he carries a disease all his life, so it really requires thought. After saying that it is the fault of the parents, we cannot say that like that, because the parents transmit a lot of things and above all life" (Interview 13). There were also expressions of pity for a child with SCD from another participant: "If it's sad because they cannot have a normal life, they cannot do everything they want. They are sick all the time so they are disabled at times. They cannot even work at times, they cannot go to see their friends at times, they are. . . . It's disabling. It's not joy. So it's serious, I think it's a serious illness. Especially since there is no cure for that" (Interview 3). A woman embedded in one organization told me that another woman much higher in a different organization infantilizes her children when she talks about them (her children were approaching their teenage years) and uses motherhood as a fulcrum to further the cause for advocating for sickle cell disease, complete with strategic crying.

One respondent said, "Someone who is carrying the trait, is saying a little 'I have an anomaly. I am not normal. And I can make children "not normal." It's not attractive'" (Interview 15). A second participant was concerned that carrier status might exacerbate existing weaknesses in the person, as if they would not be able to handle the news: "I know that there are some people who are fragile and especially those who will have a child the doubt can be brought in their head. Yes, I think it can change one's life knowing that one is carrying a disease" (Interview 12). Another participant had a more tepid, more reasoned reaction to genetic carriers for SCD: "I would be very careful with the person with whom I would make a child. It's just that you have to be careful if you have a child" (Interview 20). One woman who was a carrier stated, "We are perfectly normal, we live well. That's it, we do not have complications, and we have no sign of the disease and thank you God" (Interview 3).

One man used his partner's skin color as a determining feature of predicting carrier status, or at least gauging his own concern about it. He said, "If I put myself with a person of African descent, the question will arise much more. But if it is a person of European or Mediterranean origin, the question does not arise even if I am a carrier. But good if during the tests it turns out that I would like to know anyway. A priori you are suspicious of something, you tell yourself it's more . . .you do not think you're a carrier what. Because if my mother was more African in appearance, I might feel more concerned. You see, but on the side of my mother they are still much lighter" (Interview 2). As a dark-skinned woman, I found this comment interesting because contrary to the adage about "judging books by their cover" here was someone who felt comfortable and justified in doing exactly that.

One participant knew someone who ended his relationship so as not to have a child with sickle cell disease (Interview 17). Overall, participants did not seem to distinguish between responsibilities as men or women as potential parents, such as whether or not a woman had more responsibility to know her partners as the bearer of the children. For example, a man who had sickle cell disease used his own experience to know adamantly that he would be deliberate about preventing children with the disease. He said, "Love is important. But at what cost? I will not put a child in trouble. [Or us] too. [SCD] can break a couple too. If a relationship becomes really serious, if I really want to conceive a child with her, to make my life with her, of course. At that moment, I go to see my doctor to ask him if there is possibility. If there is possibility I leave the girl. Even if I like her, I'll leave her. For me, I do not want to make sickle cell children. Never. There are sickle cell patients who make sickle cell children, I cannot do it. I could not do it" (Interview 22).

LACK OF CONCERN FOR PEOPLE WITH SICKLE CELL DISEASE

Respondents in one-on-one interviews expressed awareness of sickle cell disease but considered themselves socially distant and therefore unconcerned about it, unless someone in their most immediate social network of closest family and friends had the disease. With respect to sickle cell disease, one participant stated, "There is a communication problem. There are people who know a lot. There is a real imbalance of information. There are people who know a lot, and people who know nothing at all" (Interview 16). This local interpretation of concern has implications for sickle cell interventions and outreach in the region. Essentially, one has to know the disease to understand it, which makes sense, but if the disease is mostly hidden, then it is not well known: "people have evolved anyway because their families have known sick children too. After that, people become more tolerant. It's ignorance that makes people talk like that. But after, as soon as they know, they know, it's okay" (Interview 22).

People are very family-oriented; they come from large families and even distant relatives are included (Interview 13). For this reason, people in Guadeloupe seem to have a finite amount of care and concern for others. As one man explained to me, "If they do not know anyone, people do not care. Frankly, people do not care, that's the word. It's not to be rude but people do not care. Frankly, people do not care. In any case, people have so much to do in a day that they will not feel sorry for this or that person. It's like that, unfortunately, but it's like that" (Interview 22). People who have the disease in their families have to create their own communities of understanding: "a little bit of a clan of patients, around which only the people really concerned, that is to say the parents, and eventually the friends who are really aware" (Interview 15).

CONCLUSIONS

This research highlights the need for analysis of the intersectional nature of people in general and in the Caribbean specifically, of race with nationality and gender and culture in order to understand how a genetic disease like sickle cell disease is interpreted in local settings. Slavery remains a powerful theme in Guadeloupe because not only is it the explanation for sickle cell disease in the region, it is also the reason why all of their ancestors came to Guadeloupe, of their own volition or not. Thus, the geography of the Caribbean is part of the explanation for the prevalence of sickle cell disease in Guadeloupe. The long legacy of slavery in Guadeloupe has recently been placed in a public light with the 2015 opening of the Memorial ACTe, a Caribbean Centre on the Expression and Memory of Slavery & the Slave Trade situated in the capital Pointe à Pitre and built on the site of a factory.

Sickle cell disease is racialized in Guadeloupe to the extent that some of the participants believed they could guess the potential for being a genetic carrier; the darker the skin tone or the higher the number of African ancestors, the higher the probability of being a carrier for SCD. Having African descent, which most people in Guadeloupe share, by this logic, has some risk for SCD. The false belief that non-Guadeloupean French people having no genetic risk for SCD plays into a racial hierarchy that whiteness is better, as some participants in these interviews shared anecdotes about people they know choosing whiter-skinned sexual partners to conceive their children. These strategies still put children at risk for being born with sickle cell disease or other hemoglobinopathies. Public health efforts need to educate communities about the fact that carriers for sickle cell disease primarily do have African descent, but they are not the only ones, and carrier status certainly cannot be determined by sight.

Because of the nature of a tense France-Guadeloupe political relationship, and the fact that the medical establishment comes from hexagonal France, local medical professionals will need to collaborate with cultural stakeholders in order to develop a screening program for adults so that they can know their carrier status simply before they engage in procreative sexual activity. Any program would need to develop as a local, Guadeloupean-led enterprise, to prevent a risk of furthering the perception that France is a patronizing force in the archipelago. The newborn screening program has been very successful, but efforts need to be placed on informing adults before they become parents. In collaboration with these cultural stakeholders, an adult screening program could decrease stigma by highlighting the high prevalence of carriers of varying skin colors and geographic origins; also, adults need to know their genetic risk as individuals, not as couples, since sexual coupling is variable and men are perceived as having more than one simultaneous partner. Screenings need to be common and mundane to be effective and accompanied by counseling about the results. As more people know their status, however, it will be important to make sure that people do not feel ashamed if they have children afflicted with SCD. More public attention to SCD would be beneficial for men and women, as long as people afflicted and affected by SCD are not exploited in the process. Through targeted health education and increasing men's participation in their own medical care, men might see that a "strong" man can be someone who takes care of his health and the health of his future children. Through these efforts, it is possible to shift Guadeloupean people into active concern about this serious disease and its consequences.

WORKS CITED

2015. "Guadeloupe: a paradise subsidized by France." *Global Property Guide*, 2015/08/25/.

Ahmad, Waqar I. U., and Karl Atkin. 1996. "Ethnicity and Caring for a Disabled Child: The Case of Children with Sickle Cell or Thalassaemia." *British Journal of Social Work* 26 (6):755–775.

Ahmed, S., J. M. Green, and J. Hewison. 2006. "Attitudes towards prenatal diagnosis and termination of pregnancy for thalassaemia in pregnant Pakistani women in the North of England." *Prenatal Diagnosis* 26 (3):248–257.

Al Arrayed, S., and A. Al Hajeri. 2010. "Public awareness of sickle cell disease in bahrain." *Annals of Saudi Medicine* 30 (4):284–288+338.

Anderson, Moji, and Monika Asnani. 2013. "'You Just Have to Live With It': Coping With Sickle Cell Disease in Jamaica." *Qualitative Health Research* 23 (5):655–664. doi: 10.1177/1049732313480048.

Arcangeli, Myriam. 2015. *Sherds of history: domestic life in colonial Guadeloupe*.

Ashenburg, Katherine. 1990. "Guadeloupe's Fresh, Fiery Creole Cuisine." *New York Times*, Apr 22, 6.

Atkin, K., S. Ahmed, J. Hewison, and J. M. Green. 2008. "Decision-making and ante-natal screening for sickle cell and Thalassaemia Disorders: To What Extent do Faith and Religious Identity Mediate Choice?" *Current Sociology* 56 (1):77–98.

Ballas, S. K., K. Gupta, and P. Adams-Graves. 2012. "Sickle cell pain: a critical reappraisal." *Blood* 120 (18):3647–56. doi: 10.1182/blood-2012-04-383430.

Bangou, Henri. 1987. *La Guadeloupe*. Paris: Editions L'Harmattan.

Bangou, Henri. 1988. *Les voies de la souveraineté: peuplement et institutions à la Guadeloupe (des origines à nos jours), Collection Parti-pris*. Paris: Éditions Caribéennes.

Bangou, Henri. 2001. *La Guadeloupe et sa décolonisation, ou, Un demi-siècle d'enfantement*. Paris: L'Harmattan.

Bediako, S. M., and C. Haywood Jr. 2009. "Sickle cell disease in a "postracial" America." *Journal of the National Medical Association* 101 (10):1065–1066.

Bediako, Shawn M., and Kimberly R. Moffitt. 2011. "Race and social attitudes about sickle cell disease." *Ethnicity & Health* 16 (4–5):423–429. doi: 10.1080/13557858.2011.552712.

Berghs, Maria, Simon M. Dyson, and Karl Atkin. 2015. "Resignifying the sickle cell gene: Narratives of genetic risk, impairment and repair." *Health:*. doi: 10.1177/1363459315595850.

Bonilla, Yarimar. 2015. *Non-sovereign futures: French Caribbean politics in the wake of disenchantment*.

Bourzac, Katherine. 2017. "Gene therapy: Erasing sickle-cell disease." *Nature* 549: S28. doi: 10.1038/549S28a.

Brennan-Cook, Jill, Emily Bonnabeau, Ravenne Aponte, Christina Augustin, and Paula Tanabe. 2018. "Barriers to Care for Persons With Sickle Cell Disease: The Case Manager's Opportunity to Improve Patient Outcomes." *Professional Case Management* 23 (4):213–219. doi: 10.1097/ncm.0000000000000260.

Brown, Shan-Estelle, Daniel F Weisberg, and William H Sledge. 2015. "Family caregiving for adults with sickle cell disease and extremely high hospital use." *Journal of Health Psychology*. doi: 10.1177/1359105315588215.

Carter, Bob, and Simon M Dyson. 2011. "Territory, Ancestry and Descent: The Politics of Sickle Cell Disease." *Sociology* 45 (6):963–976. doi: 10.1177/0038038511416159.

Ciribassi, Rebekah M., and Crystal L. Patil. 2016. "'We don't wear it on our sleeve': Sickle cell disease and the (in)visibile body in parts." *Social Science & Medicine* 148:131–8. doi: http://dx.doi.org/10.1016/j.socscimed.2015.11.033.

Ducrocq, R., M. Benkerrou, L. Brahimi, M. Belloy, M. L. Briard, E. Vilmer, and J. Elion. 2001. "Neonatal screening for sickle cell disease: evaluation of a five-year experience in the northern part of the Paris area." *Archives De Pediatrie* 8 (5):474–480.

Dyson, S. M., K. Atkin, L. A. Culley, S. E. Dyson, H. Evans, and D. T. Rowley. 2010. "Disclosure and sickle cell disorder: A mixed methods study of the young person with sickle cell at school." *Social Science and Medicine* 70 (12):2036–2044.

Emerson, Robert M., Rachel I. Fretz, and Linda L. Shaw. 1995. *Writing ethnographic fieldnotes, Chicago guides to writing, editing, and publishing*: Chicago: University of Chicago Press.

Ettorre, Elizabeth. 2002. "A critical look at the new genetics: conceptualizing the links between reproduction, gender and bodies." *Critical Public Health* 12 (3):237–250.

Feagin, Joe, and Zinobia Bennefield. 2014. "Systemic racism and U.S. health care." *Social Science & Medicine* 103:7–14. doi: http://dx.doi.org/10.1016/j.socscimed.2013.09.006.

Frampton, Susan Barbara. 1990. *Applied anthropology and public policy: the study of the Hartford Newborn Sickle Cell Screening Pilot Project*.

Fullwiley, Duana. 2004. "Discriminate biopower and everyday biopolitics: views on sickle cell testing in Dakar." *Medical Anthropology* 23 (2):157–194.

Fullwiley, Duana. 2010. "Revaluating genetic causation: Biology, economy, and kinship in Dakar, Senegal." *American Ethnologist* 37 (4):638–661.

Fullwiley, Duana. 2012. *The enculturated gene: sickle cell health politics and biological difference in West Africa*. Princeton: Princeton University Press.

Galacteros, F. 1996. "Neonatal screening for sickle cell disease in metropolitan France." *Archives De Pédiatrie* 3 (10):1026–1031.

Glassberg, Jeffrey A., Paula Tanabe, Annie Chow, Katrina Harper, Carlton Haywood Jr, Michael R. DeBaun, and Lynne D. Richardson. 2013. "Emergency Provider Analgesic Practices and Attitudes Toward Patients With Sickle Cell Disease." *Annals of Emergency Medicine* (0). doi: http://dx.doi.org/10.1016/j.annemergmed.2013.02.004.

Glassberg, Jeffrey, Paula Tanabe, Lynne Richardson, and Michael DeBaun. 2013. "Among emergency physicians, use of the term 'Sickler' is associated with negative attitudes toward people with sickle cell disease." *American Journal of Hematology* 88 (6):532–533. doi: 10.1002/ajh.23441.

Grossman, L. K., N. A. Holtzman, E. Charney, and A. D. Schwartz. 1985. "Neonatal screening and genetic counseling for sickle cell trait." *American Journal Of Diseases Of Children (1960)* 139 (3):241–244.

Handwerker, W. Penn. 2002. *Quick ethnography*. Walnut Creek, CA: AltaMira Press.

Haywood Jr, C., S. Lanzkron, N. Ratanawongsa, S. M. Bediako, L. Lattimer, N. R. Powe, and M. C. Beach. 2010. "The association of provider communication with trust among adults with sickle cell disease." *Journal of General Internal Medicine* 25 (6):543–548.

Haywood Jr, Carlton, Paula Tanabe, Rakhi Naik, Mary Catherine Beach, and Sophie Lanzkron. 2013. "The impact of race and disease on sickle cell patient wait times in the emergency department." *The American Journal of Emergency Medicine* 31 (4):651–656. doi: http://dx.doi.org/10.1016/j.ajem.2012.11.005.

Helman, Cecil. 2000. *Culture, health, and illness*. 4th ed. Oxford; Boston: Butterworth-Heinemann.

Lanzkron, Sophie, C. Patrick Carroll, and Carlton Haywood. 2013. "Mortality Rates and Age at Death from Sickle Cell Disease: U.S., 1979–2005." *Public Health Reports* 128 (2):110–116.

Lieberman, Leonard, and Rodney C. Kirk. 2004. "What Should We Teach about the concept of Race?" *Anthropology & Education Quarterly* 35 (1):137–145. doi: 10.1525/aeq.2004.35.1.137.

Maddox, Camee. 2015. "'Yes We Can! Down with Colonization!' Race, Gender, and the 2009 General Strike in Martinique." *Transforming Anthropology* 23 (2):90–103. doi: doi:10.1111/traa.12047.

Managan, Kathe. 2012. "Words to Make you Laugh?: Performing the Public in Guadeloupean Comedy Sketches." *Journal of Linguistic Anthropology* 22 (2):E83-E104. doi: 10.1111/j.1548-1395.2012.01149.x.

Managan, Kathe. 2015. "'One Hand Washes the Other': Social Capital and the Politics of Leisure in Guadeloupean Associations." *French Politics, Culture & Society* 33 (3):74–94. doi: 10.3167/fpcs.2015.330304.

Mann, Monica. 2010. "Pain, Personhood, and Translating Sickle Cell Anemia." *Transforming Anthropology* 18 (2):146–150.

Rapp, Rayna. 1997. "Communicating about chromosomes: patients, providers, and cultural assumptions." *Journal of the American Medical Women's Association* 52 (1):28–9, 32.

Rapp, Rayna. 1998. "Refusing Prenatal Diagnosis: The Meanings of Bioscience in a Multicultural World." *Science, Technology, & Human Values* 23 (1):45–70.

Rouse, Carolyn Moxley. 2009. *Uncertain suffering: racial health care disparities and sickle cell disease*. Berkeley: University of California Press.

Savas, N., E. Turhan, T. Inandi, and H. Kaya. 2010. "Hemoglobinopathy awareness among high school students in Antakya (Antioch), Turkey." *International Journal of Hematology* 91 (3):413–418.

Schneider, Paul. 2006. "French, and Beach, Spoken Here." *New York Times*, 2006/02/05/.

Segal, Jodi B., and Johns Hopkins University Evidence-based Practice Center. 2008. *Hydroxyurea for the treatment of sickle cell disease*. Rockville, Md.: Agency for Healthcare Research and Quality.

Shanklin, Eugenia. 2000. "Representations of Race and Racism in American Anthropology." *Current Anthropology* 41 (1):99–103. doi: 10.1086/300105.

Talano, J. A., and M. S. Cairo. 2015. "Hematopoietic stem cell transplantation for sickle cell disease: state of the science." *Eur J Haematol* 94 (5):391–9. doi: 10.1111/ejh.12447.

Tanabe, P., J. Porter, M. Creary, E. Kirkwood, S. Miller, E. Ahmed-Williams, and K. Hassell. 2010. "A qualitative analysis of best self-management practices: sickle cell disease." *J Natl Med Assoc* 102 (11):1033–41.

Tapper, Melbourne. 1999. *In the blood: sickle cell anemia and the politics of race*. Philadelphia: University of Pennsylvania Press.

Tarer, Vanessa, Maryse Etienne-Julan, Jean-Pierre Diara, Marie Sylvaine Belloy, Martin Mukizi-Mukaza, Jacques Elion, and Marc Romana. 2006. "Sickle cell anemia in Guadeloupean children: pattern and prevalence of acute clinical events." *European Journal of Haematology* 76 (3):193–199.

Wailoo, Keith. 2001. *Dying in the city of the blues: sickle cell anemia and the politics of race and health*. Chapel Hill: University of North Carolina Press.

Wallraff, Barbara. 2002. A Secret Caribbean. *The Atlantic*, February 2002.

Weisberg, D., G. Balf-Soran, W. Becker, S. E. Brown, and W. Sledge. 2013. "I'm talking about pain": sickle cell disease patients with extremely high hospital use." *Journal of Hospital Medicine* 8 (1):42–6. doi: 10.1002/jhm.1987.

Wille, M. C., B. Weitz, P. Kerper, and S. Frazier. 2004. "Advances in preconception genetic counseling." *The Journal of perinatal & neonatal nursing* 18 (1):28–40.

Wong, Trisha E., Amanda M. Brandow, Wendy Lim, and Richard Lottenberg. 2014. "Update on the use of hydroxyurea therapy in sickle cell disease." *Blood* 124 (26):3850–3857. doi: 10.1182/blood-2014-08-435768.

Zempsky, W. T. 2009. "Treatment of sickle cell pain: fostering trust and justice." *JAMA* 302 (22):2479–80. doi: 10.1001/jama.2009.1811.

Chapter Six

Convergent Therapies in Peru's Amazon

Enriching Mental Wellness through Ayahuasca and Psychotherapy

Olivia Marcus and Evgenia Fotiou

This chapter considers the implications of the transnational movement of clients and practitioners who seek to find therapeutic outcomes with traditional Amazonian healing techniques in Peru. In particular, growing interest in ayahuasca, a psychedelic tea that purportedly confers a range of therapeutic benefits, attracts people from all corners of the globe to urban and remote regions of the jungle. The healing techniques and technologies of the shamans of the Peruvian Amazon are, of course, not static practices and beliefs unchanged over centuries; rather they are dynamic and constantly changing practices embedded within indigenous cosmologies that developed amidst pre-colonial interactions among indigenous societies and have been subsequently affected by over 500 years of colonial influences that include Christian missions, forced conversions, indigenous enslavement, the rubber boom of the early twentieth century, logging and mining, narco-trafficking, oil extraction, and tourism. Over the past couple of decades, local healing practices are being affected by an influx of foreigners who seek shamanic healing techniques. Traditional Amazonian medicine (TAM) is increasingly offered with an assortment of other techniques ranging from psychotherapy to acupuncture, Reiki, Ayurveda, yoga, sweat lodges (*temascales)*, and cacao ceremonies, among others.

This chapter takes particular interest in the growing relationship between Western theories and styles of psychotherapy as tools for facilitating the healing process among people who seek mental wellness through shamanic healing in the Amazon. We begin with a background on the "traditional" uses of ayahuasca in Peru, popularly referred to as ayahuasca shamanism or *curanderismo*. We then explore the implications of new uses of the tea in the study of global mental health. Finally, we consider the state of therapeutic pluralism in Peru's Amazon, where ethnographic data enriches an understanding of the use of various modes of healing for improved spiritual or mental well-being.

CURANDERISMO IN THE UPPER PERUVIAN AMAZON

Ayahuasca (*Banisteropsis caapi*) is a Quechua-language name for a jungle liana that grows in parts of the Amazon rainforest that span Peru, Brazil, Ecuador, Colombia, Bolivia, and Venezuela. When mixed with the leaves of either chacruna (*Psychotria viridis*) or chaliponga (*Diplopterys cabrerana*) and boiled down for hours, the result is a psychoactive tea that often has strong visionary and purgative effects.[1] Other admixtures may include wild Amazonian tobacco (*Nicotiana rustica*) and *toé* (*Brugmansia sauveolens)*, though some people prepare the tea with over fifteen different plants. For centuries, ritual uses of the ayahuasca vine have been practiced by select indigenous peoples in the Amazon forest for healing, auguring events, hunting, and telepathic communication across distances (Dobkin de Rios 1972; Luna 1986; Harner 1972). In some preparations, just the vine itself is boiled down into a highly purgative tea that has its own salubrious properties (Torres Romero 2012). In the Peruvian Amazon, ayahuasca is traditionally prepared and served by a *curandero (*a healer) or *vegetalista* (someone with specialized knowledge of plants), though both terms are often used interchangeable with "shaman" in common parlance (Luna 1986). Among Peruvian *curanderos*, ayahuasca is not traditionally used in isolation but in conjunction with a pharmacopeia of medicinal plants (*vegetales*) and other diagnostic and therapeutic techniques such as plant diets, plant baths, pulse reading, tonics, and lifestyle prescriptions. The process known as a "plant diet" (*la dieta)* is integral to Peruvian *curanderismo* as a means for people to heal and/or learn from the plants through fasting, food restrictions (e.g., no salt, sugar, pork, ice, or alcohol), social isolation, drinking plant tonics, and bathing in preparations of prescribed plants. The diagnostic process often occurs before a ceremony, though ceremonies also enable a *curandero* to assess the well-being of participants. A ceremonial participant does not need to drink ayahuasca in order for the healing ritual to be effective; indeed, before the influx of foreign clientele, it was rather uncommon for anyone but the *curandero* to drink ayahuasca.

While the medicinal potential of ayahuasca is often emphasized in contemporary shamanic practices, it should be noted that many indigenous uses of ayahuasca have never been for healing, but are used among shamans or in collective rituals for other purposes (Gow 1992). In indigenous contexts, *dietas* may be used as a rite of passage from adolescence into adulthood; as a training process for *curanderos* or *vegetalistas*; or to fortify the body and mind for improved physical strength, immune function, and sexual performance (Sanz-Biset & Cañigueral 2011). A significant feature of *curanderismo* that is often overlooked in the literature is the learning and invocation of *icaros*, which are songs used to call the spirit of the plants during the preparation of plant medicines; upon administration of the remedy; during an ayahuasca ceremony; and during a plant diet. The number of *icaros* that a shaman knows and the respective power of each *icaro* is a potent indication of the practitioner's abilities and knowledge of healing and/or sorcery, since *icaros* represent their direct contact with the spirit world. In an apprenticeship, a *curandero* will teach his or her student some *icaros*, though apprentices are supposed to receive their own *icaros* through direct communication with the spirit of the plants. Individuals often receive *icaros* through *dietas*, during ayahuasca ceremonies, and in dreams (Luna 1986; Beyer 2009).

MENTAL HEALTH AND PLANT MEDICINE

A growing international clientele is attracted to Peru's Amazon to try ayahuasca for its medicinal potential, for spiritual development, or through simple curiosity (Dobkin de Rios 1994; Lewis 2008; Fotiou 2010; Homan 2017). The emphasis on its salubrious effects by westerners has brought increased attention to ayahuasca ceremonies for the treatment of mental health conditions, notably anxiety and depression (Osório et al. 2015; Sanches et al. 2016), trauma/PTSD (Nielson & Megler 2012), addiction rehabilitation (Mabit 2007; Thomas et al. 2013; Berlowitz et al. 2017), protracted grief (González et al. 2017), and eating disorders (Lefrance et al. 2017). The preoccupation with global mental health has emerged as a top public health priority over the past two decades due to the rising prevalence of mental illness and the associated social and economic toll (Becker & Kleinman 2013; Becker et al. 2013). In a recent update, Vigo and colleagues (2016) reported that the global burden of mental illness accounts for 32.4 percent of years lived with disability (YLDs) and 13.0 percent of disability-adjusted life-years (DALYs)—almost a third more than previously estimated in 2013. Among the top twenty causes of the global burden of disease, major depression ranks as number two, anxiety disorders at seven, schizophrenia at eleven, dysthymia (persistent mild depression) at sixteen, and bipolar at seventeen, which places mental illness as a "distant first in the global burden of disease in terms of YLDs" (Vigo et al. 2016, 171). In the United States, the financial burden of mental illness is estimated at $300 billion annually and is expected to increase over the next twenty years (Insel 2009). The application of traditional Amazonian medicine, namely *dietas* and ayahuasca ceremonies, for the improvement of mental wellness may be a potent resource for addressing the burden of mental health.

While ayahuasca and other medicinal plants are traditionally used to treat specific physical illnesses such as parasites, infections, cancers, arthritic and rheumatic symptoms, autoimmune conditions, and respiratory problems, within Amazonian cosmology the physical and psycho-spiritual are not disentangled into their respective "types" of illness or wellness. The body, spirit, nature, and cosmos are parts of one whole, of which each aspect needs care and attention for the well-being of the others. Still, the expertise in plant use among *curanderos* in Peru has traditionally been used to improve mental health and address psychosomatic disorders. For example, in a decade-long study among healers in Northern Peru, ethnobotanist Rainier Bussman (2013) found that out of 510 commonly used plant medicines, 98 (19.1 percent) are used specifically for psychosomatic and nervous system problems.

In contrast to the integrated cosmology of Amazonian peoples, the Western biomedical approach to mental health silos the psychological from that of the social or physical, unless put into combined categories of "psychosocial" or "psychosomatic" illnesses. The U.S. National Institute of Mental Health recognizes mental illness as a brain disorder marked by abnormal brain activity (Insel 2009). Conventional psychiatry conjures diagnoses through statistical inference, offering a satellite of characteristic symptoms to describe various mood disorders, personality disorders, traumatic disorders, and phobias. These diagnostic categories are, of course, quite useful for the identification and treatment of adverse psychiatric or psychological conditions, as well as for surveying populations for their prevalence. In this psychiatric model of care, diagnostic strategies and treatment options remain limited and serve to reinforce the distinction between individual and society, body and mind. This is perhaps the most important distinction between Amazonian healing practices and conventional psychiatry: the former situates the individual within a world of spirits, ancestors, and living brethren with whom they are connected and who affect the individual's health. The etiology of illness in Amazonian cosmology goes beyond the individual, thus the treatment must as well. Yet when westerners enter this world of healing, they bring with them the rigid principles of a brain-based model of mental health, one in which abnormal patterns of brain activity must be "corrected" in order to achieve mental wellness, often through pharmaceutical or behavioral intervention. In ayahuasca ceremonies, however, participants often experience altered states of consciousness in which they may have numinous experiences, speak with spirits, encounter dead relatives or ancestors, or revisit past traumas. The ceremony itself may be overwhelming, confusing, ecstatic, and certainly deeply therapeutic if properly prepared for and integrated.

The integration of experiences with altered states of consciousness is a prominent concern among the therapeutic community who acknowledge ayahuasca, among other psychedelic substances, to have potent therapeutic value (Loizaga-Velder & Verres 2014). From the international therapeutic community comprised of Western-trained mental health workers, traditional shamans, and neo-shamans has emerged an ongoing dialogue between Western psychology and Amazonian cosmology in which therapeutic forms converge and mutually influence how clients and practitioners perceive illness, wellness, and healing. In a qualitative study among indigenous healers and Western-trained therapists who use ayahuasca in the treatment of addiction, Loizaga-Velder and Verres (2014) found that practitioners considered integration to be integral for long-term positive therapeutic outcomes. The term "psychedelic integration therapy" is now a popular topic at scientific conferences, on retreat center websites, and among the therapeutic community. The advent of certification programs for "psychedelic coaches" or "psychedelic-assisted therapies," as well as workshops that offer continuing education credits for training in psychedelic-related clinical practice are part of the growing institutionalization of what has for many decades been a fringe practice. These trainings and accreditations also indicate the perception among mental health workers of the critical role of psychotherapeutic intervention with the use of psychedelics.

AYAHUASCA RETREAT CENTERS: IQUITOS AND TARAPOTO

A proliferation of ayahuasca healing centers in Peru nourishes the ongoing therapeutic pluralism present in urban and peri-urban spaces of Peru's Amazon, where biomedicine, traditional Chinese medicine, Ayurveda, yoga, Reiki, and traditional Amazonian medicine are on offer. The number of these centers can only be estimated, for there are no regulatory measures that necessitate registry as an "ayahuasca center" or "traditional healing center." Anyone from any nationality can buy land, build a center, build a website, and start recruiting customers. In this chapter we focus on two regions of the Northwest Amazon, San Martín and Loreto, where the two authors have conducted ethnographic fieldwork.[2] In Loreto, and particularly in the areas surrounding Iquitos and Nauta, ayahuasca has become a main attraction for tourists and travelers. The number of people who have poured into Iquitos on a quest for the brew has risen dramatically since the first few years of the twenty-first century, from approximately 200 per year in 2005 to some estimated thousands per year by 2015 (Fotiou 2016). Some of these people come for eco-tourism and find themselves intrigued by the mysterious and potent tea, while many others come specifically seeking a shaman with which to drink ayahuasca or do a *dieta*. Ethnographer and journalist Carlos Suarez-Álvarez (2017) estimates that in 2016 there were at least forty known ayahuasca retreat centers functioning in and around Iquitos. This estimate does not include the many shamans who work independently from their homes or from more secluded places in the forest. Suarez-Álvarez visited ten of these centers, which collectively estimated that about 4,000 people had come to their centers in the past year, staying for approximately seven to ten days, but sometimes two to three weeks or even several months. If we were to multiply this by four to make a rough estimate among the forty known centers just in Iquitos, he suggests there are *at least* 16,000 ayahuasca-related visitors in one small region in just one year.

The city of Tarapoto, which is the commercial center of San Martín, is an urban center located in the Amazonian highlands, where the Andean mountain range meets the forest to create the *ceja de selva* (high jungle). Tarapoto is smaller than Iquitos, and until recent years its development remained much slower. Iquitos is considered the "gateway to the Amazon," a popular tourist destination for seeing wildlife, visiting indigenous villages, and buying local crafts. Before it became a tourist destination, however, Iquitos was an early colonial center in the Amazon and the nucleus of the rubber boom of the 1920s. During this time, a community of wealthy rubber barons built elegant hotels, cafés, churches, and even an opera house in the central part of the city, creating a strange metropolitan aesthetic the remnants of which can still be detected among the urban decay that has given way to a more rustic appearance. Tarapoto, on the other hand, remained a lonely backwater that sits along the Mayo and Huallaga rivers, hundreds of miles southwest of Iquitos. During the 1980s, the Huallaga Valley became the world's most intensive site of coca production, as well as an outpost for the violent Marxist-Maoist organization Shining Path (*Sendero Luminoso)*, and a point of contact for narco-traffickers, making it a rather dangerous place for travelers. Nevertheless, a trickling of intrepid foreigners would come through the region to see the beautiful waterfalls and lagunas, hike the cloud forest, visit local Lamista communities, or take a bus to the nearby tourist destinations of Moyobamba and Chachapoyas. The scale of coca production dramatically reduced by the early 2000s and Tarapoto has become a peaceful city with a rapidly growing tourism industry. Even so, the region is still affected by subsequent economic booms in oil extraction, illegal logging, bioprospecting, and ecotourism.

In San Martín, the first ayahuasca healing centers designed for a non-local demographic began opening near Tarapoto in the early 1990s. The oldest and most well known of these centers is the Takiwasi Center for Addiction

Rehabilitation and Research on Traditional Medicines (*Takiwasi Centro de Rehabilitación de Toxicómanos y de Investigación de Medicinas Tradicionales*). Established in 1992 by a French medical doctor and a Peruvian medical doctor with a multidisciplinary team of psychologists, biochemical researchers, and *curanderos*, the center is designed to create a bridge between Western biomedical epistemologies of healing and those of traditional Amazonian peoples in order to best treat drug addiction, particularly misuse of alcohol and crack/cocaine, which became an epidemic problem in the region due to narco-trafficking and civil conflict from the 1980s through the early 2000s. Takiwasi is not a retreat center, but a therapeutic community and mental health clinic recognized by the Peruvian Ministry of Health, where ayahuasca ceremonies, *dieta*s, plant baths, and other rituals are complemented by psychotherapy. As a research center, they have also supported publications on the efficacy of their therapeutic approach (Mabit 2007; Mabit & Sieber 2006; Horák 2014; Berlowitz 2017). Takiwasi began as a project to address serious substance abuse and mental health issues in San Martín, yet the center is an all-male therapeutic community, which means that females cannot intern themselves as long-term patients. This is a legal issue: in Peru, therapeutic communities cannot be co-gender, so Takiwasi would have to build a separate center to host female inpatients, which would put a great financial burden on the existing clinic. It was explained to Olivia that Takiwasi is a "pilot" project, meant to provide a proof of concept that other people can use as a model for starting similar projects. Thus, if another group wanted to create a community for females, that would be a supported initiative. However, one of the therapists also suggested a caveat: that women in the area cannot commit as readily to a nine-month inpatient program as men do because of their "family responsibilities." Others have suggested that there simply is not enough female clientele to sustain such a project. The validity of these arguments is difficult to assess without a detailed study, but there is certainly one glaring issue: that a large portion of clients at Takiwasi are from foreign countries, mainly Central/South American and European, and a large portion of Peruvians come from well-off families in Lima. This leaves open the question of whether there might indeed be demand for an all-female inpatient facility, at least among foreign clientele. But Takiwasi does not exclude women. The clinic is open to females who want to come for a *dieta* and the therapists see outpatients who either travel from surrounding towns or do Skype sessions from other countries.

In addition to Takiwasi, other ayahuasca healing centers around Tarapoto began to open in the 1990s, but most have emerged on the scene in the past ten to fifteen years, particularly in the past five. Over the course of her fieldwork in the area, Olivia estimates there to be at least twenty-nine ayahuasca retreat centers that span the areas of Tarapoto, Lamas, San Roque de Cumbaza, San Antonio de Cumbaza, Pamashto, Sauce, and Chazuta. Most of these centers are owned either by non-Peruvians or non-local Peruvians (i.e., from Lima or other parts of the country), thus this estimate does not include the many local shamans who work independently in their communities. The prices of these retreat centers range from 620 USD to 900 USD for a seven-day retreat; 1250 USD to 2689 USD for a fourteen-day retreat; and can reach up to 3,000–4,000 USD for a month. Prices vary depending on the privacy of the room, length of stay, and availability of other services (e.g., Ayurvedic treatments, energy healings, massage, yoga retreats, crystal healing). Five of these centers claim to have psychologists on staff to aid clientele during their diets, and one offers daily integration circles. Most *curanderos* in this region are male, which can largely be attributed to local gender norms concerning division of labor: women are expected to look after their family and children, and therefore often do not have the flexibility to do the months and years of *dietas* that are necessary for training as a *curandero*. Nevertheless, *curanderas* do exist in the area, though the female shamans that Olivia did come across tended to be well-educated and often from foreign countries (e.g., France, Czech Republic, Australia) or from other parts of Peru (e.g., Pucallpa, Lima, Ayacucho).

THE CONVERGENCE OF SHAMANISM AND PSYCHOTHERAPY

As the numbers of ayahuasca retreat centers and their clientele increase, so does the interest in providing some sort of therapeutic integration process. This arises for two main reasons: first, many people come to seek alternative mental health treatment and therefore arrive at these centers with psychiatric conditions (e.g., major depression, PTSD, eating disorders) for which they may have been taking potent medications. Those with pre-existing psychiatric conditions may benefit greatly by seeking pre-trip advice and follow-up with a professional who comes from the cultural context of the client. The popularity of ayahuasca for the treatment of depression, trauma/PTSD, and anxiety is reflected in the ethnographic and psychological literature (e.g., Winkleman 2005; Schmidt et al., 2010; Kavenská & Simonová 2015; Cohen 2017), as well as in popular media.[3] Kavenská and Simonová (2015) found that among seventy-seven people who came to the Peruvian Amazon to drink ayahuasca, a third reported doing so for mental health benefits. Similarly, in his study conducted at a retreat center outside of Iquitos, Cohen (2017) learned that ten of thirteen participants had a traumatic experience that influenced their decision to drink ayahuasca. While an integration process is suggested for any person undertaking a process with ayahuasca, it is arguably more critical among people who seek ayahuasca specifically for mental health issues.

Second, and related, the processes involved in drinking ayahuasca and other medicinal plants often evoke intense emotional states that may need some intervention for psychologically integrating life-changing experiences that may upend an individual's worldview or sense of self (Lewis 2008; Ray & Lassiter 2016). While this process is necessarily built into the protocol at Takiwasi, where it has been put into practice for over twenty-five years, other centers are in the process of building up a best-practice scenario. Many metropolitan Peruvians seek out ayahuasca healing alongside other Central, South, and North American, European, East- and South-East Asian clientele. Some will attend retreat centers, while others seek out independent shamans. Considering the range in cultural background among clientele, defining what the process of integration is and how to go about it becomes a matter of debate.

Integration connotes a process that begins before the ayahuasca ceremony or plant diet, ideally before a person decides to embark on a shamanic healing experience. Traditionally, ayahuasca is taken in a ritual context, often among family or community members and with a shaman who will guide them in preparation for the ceremony and in interpreting the experience. The process of integration is embedded in the indigenous cultural context and therefore a structure for psychointegration based on Western theoretical concepts in psychology is often neither appropriate nor necessary. The non-local person, on the other hand, generally lacks this infrastructure and awareness of the Amazonian cosmology in which ayahuasca shamanism is embedded, thus some preparation in terms of cultural difference is recommended, while psychological and physiological preparation should be considered critical to beneficial outcomes (Shanon 2002; Ray & Lassiter 2016). Yet it is after (and sometimes during) the ceremony or diet when integration therapy is most common, sometimes manifesting as a group-sharing process or as individual psychotherapy sessions. As one informant, a psychedelic integration coach in the United States, put it:

> To me, medicine work is not the time that's actually spent on the medicine. Medicines are catalyst for change, but the change happens once the ceremony is over. So, integration is that time spent integrating the insides and the lessons from the psychedelic realm into everyday life. Into our daily life. Utilizing them in daily practices, building upon the insights that were learned . . . concentrating on the spiritual aspect, the physical aspect, the emotional aspect, the lifestyle, the mental state . . . relationships. So, there are five life domains, basically five domains that can potentially all get highly affected by medicine work. So it's paying a lot of attention to making sure that they're all balanced following the psychedelic experience. (April 2017)

As an emergent praxis among Western-trained mental health workers—whether clinical psychologists, social workers, psychotherapists, or mental health coaches—integration therapy has a goal to help people process their psychedelic experience to heighten therapeutic potential and self-growth. Rather than its own "style" of psychotherapy, it would best be described as a trending term for a practice within a longstanding tradition of psychedelic psychotherapy[4] that draws on theory and techniques from Jungian analytic psychology, Gestalt therapy, transpersonal psychology, mind-body practices, and the psychology of "spiritual emergence" (Grof & Grof 1989; Grob 1994; Mabit et al. 1996). At the Takiwasi clinic, the model of care is fashioned as a "therapeutic tripod": a combination of work with the plants, psychotherapy, and *convivencia* (cohabitation as a therapeutic community), all of which are integral components for the process of rehabilitation. When asked whether one component of the tripod was more important, one member of the therapeutic team responded:

> The importance is they work together. How do they work together? [long pause]. The visions that the patients have in diets, ayahuasca, tends to be in some order similar, related to the contents that the patient has in their dreams and in their psychotherapy, and in their *convivencia*. . . . So, you're working different levels through the plants, through the convivencia, and through the psychotherapy. But, it tends to be the same in different situations.
>
> . . . For example, a patient that has problems with communication will [find it] difficult to work with other people, because he cannot express what he needs, he can be upset [and] when he is really upset, he is unable to put a limit [i.e., set boundaries]. And maybe their dreams and their session of psychotherapy reveal the same situation, in the context of psychotherapy. And maybe the curanderos start to see that he has a problem in his, in his energetic center of communication, hm? And he starts to work with the plant that is useful for that purpose. And in his story of life he can recognize some stuff that is related to communication. So at all the levels you find the same, more or less. (August 2015)

In this narrative, the therapist explains that each component of the therapeutic tripod helps to integrate the others. The work with the plants, which includes ayahuasca sessions, plant diets, taking purgative plants (*purgas*), and daily low-concentration plant tonics (*plantas de contención*), helps to work through content that comes up in psychotherapy sessions, but also to evoke psychotherapeutic content that may have not come up otherwise. Similarly, the experience of *convivencia* both elicits content and helps patients to integrate their personal psychotherapeutic and plant-based work through daily interactions with fellow patients. In interviews with inpatients (five males) and with people who come for the ten-day diets (three female, two male), all informants noted the augmenting effect of the plant work on their therapeutic relationships.

Much scholarship has focused on the healing aspects of shamanism, recognizing the therapeutic potential of symbolic healing and experiences of psychological catharsis (DuBois 2011). Anthropologists have long written about the supposed similarities and differences between the shaman and the psychotherapist or psychiatrist. Early anthropologists such as Alfred Kroeber (1940), George Devereux (1956), and Weston La Barre (1972) characterized the shaman as psychotic or likened entry into shamanic trance to schizophrenic states. Others, however, have argued against the shaman-as-mentally-ill interpretation and instead advocate for a shaman-as-psychotherapist analogy, considering the shaman as a sort of specialist whose techniques can inform psychotherapeutic practice (e.g., Kiev 1968; Kakar 1982; Noll 1983, Metzner 1998; Dobkin de Rios 2002). Claude Lévi-Strauss (1963) has perhaps been most influential in his description of the parallels between psychoanalysis and shamanism, emphasizing the important role of myth and symbols in the healing process. In *The Effectiveness of Symbols,* he explains that the shaman and the analyst provide a language of symbols that allows the patient to express previously inexpressible unconscious material. Through retrieving this unconscious material for conscious use, individuals can create a harmony between myth and action (Lévi-Strauss 1963). However, he argues, there is an important difference between analyst and shaman: the shaman works within a collective orientation while the analyst must help the Western patient construct an *individual* myth.

The distinction between collectivist and individualist ethos with respect to indigenous and "modern" or "Westernized" societies has been met with resistance by some anthropologists. In a study among Hindu-Buddhist mystics in Sri Lanka, Gananath Obeyesekere (1981) seems to challenge the distinction between the individual and social myth, instead arguing that individual-psychological symbols always have a reciprocal relationship with the public, culturally sanctioned role of the symbol. Considering the Peruvian Amazon as a transnational therapeutic landscape—that is, a place where authentic healing processes occur—it may stand to reason that what at first glance appear to be "pilgrims" or "tourists" from highly individualized occidental cultures (Fotiou 2010), are not so psychologically individualized as mainstream thought might lead us to believe. Alex Gearin (2016) contributes an insightful argument against the common assumption that contemporary alternative spiritualities are individualistic, self-fulfilling pursuits that lack communal values or commitment to communal goals. In describing the use of ayahuasca among Australians as a New Age practice, he takes note that there seems to be an "orthodoxy" among many scholars that New Age spirituality, neo-shamanism included, tends to be inherently individualistic. Gearin makes the important observation that the dividual/individual binary does not apply neatly to all indigenous/modern-capitalist societies, respectively, and particularly not to all facets of these societies. Rather, he proposes that individualism and relationalism may be "integrated conceptual tool[s]" rather than opposites (Gearin 2016, 203).

Nevertheless, there exist cultural biases within traditional psychological services such that conventional Western psychotherapy focuses on the "independence and individuality in relationships, direct verbal communication styles, emotional expressiveness, clear distinctions between the mind and body, [and] intrapsychic processes in the context of mental health relationships" (Constantine et al. 2004, 112). Lewis-Fernández and Kleinman (1994) described three culture-bound assumptions in Western psychology: egocentricity (as opposed to *allocentric* or *interdependent*); Cartesian mind-body dualism; and culture as an "arbitrary phenomenon superimposed on a uniform biological reality" (Constantine et al. 2004, 113). In the cross-pollination between shamanism and psychology that has been called "psychologizing the religious," or using the cosmos as a tool for "therapizing the psyche" (Vitebsky 2003, 287), specifically in the dialogue between Western clients and their ayahuasca shamans, many of these concepts continue to be invoked, namely direct verbal communication, emotional expressiveness, and intrapsychic processes à la biochemical models of mental health. In what has been noted as the "psychologization" of ayahuasca—and shamanism in general—the ayahuasca experience is used as a form of improving self-knowledge, often by working through trauma via interpretation of unconscious or suppressed psychic content that is evoked in dreams or as visions during ceremonies (Labate 2014). Others of these biases, however, give way to narratives of seeing the body as a whole organism, interrelated not only with the psycho-spiritual, but also with the intergenerational (Mabit 2007). The notion of working out the traumas of one's ancestors or community is a significant aspect of indigenous shamanism that translates well to "modern" bodies, among whom the language of trauma is a relevant construction of the psychological self (Mabit 2007; Theidon 2014).

Over the decades, Western-oriented participants in shamanic ceremonies have changed the construction of the shaman, and ayahuasca shamanism in particular, into a practitioner who helps clients construct and take action within their individual myth (Labate 2014; Brabec de Mori 2014; Kavenská & Simonová 2015). At Centro Takiwasi, it was found that the adjunct of psychotherapy was a very welcome difference between the clinic and other ayahuasca centers. Several informants noted the lack of "professionalism" in other places, where people are allowed into ceremonies without any background checks concerning their mental health or follow-ups. One informant at Takiwasi, a twenty-nine-year-old female from Australia, remarked on her frustration with such centers:

> But what I had found is that it's, with the ayahuasca anyway . . . it wasn't very personalized. I never kind of sat with the facilitators and said "look, this is what's going on in my life, these are the issues, this is what I'm here for," you know? I just didn't feel like I was really getting anywhere. I was having very physical ceremonies, as in just purging the entire session. Like vomiting, mucus, a lot of energy moving . . . it was really frustrating, you know? Because obviously this time I had come with some expectations of what ayahuasca would be like. And just not being able to engage with someone and get feedback, you know, from a professional and someone that's kind of heard it and seen it all. (July 2015)

This client had come to do a ten-day diet with Takiwasi, having sat in many ceremonies in other parts of Peru. She suffered from intense depressive episodes and had a history of sexual trauma, which were key issues she wanted to work through using ayahuasca. When I asked why she thought the experience with Takiwasi was different from drinking ayahuasca at other centers, she was enthusiastic about the combination of psychology with the plant diet.

> Coming here, to work with a trained psychologist and my experience with J*** [her therapist]—very, very good. I've seen a few psychologists in my time and we went places in the few days that we've had our relationship, really was looking like a ten-day kind of client-psych relationship, we've gone to places that I've not gone with other psychs, working with them longer. . . . The dieta, the plants, the solitude. Yeah, it's just a very unique, affective combination. At least for me, because I've gone to other psychs and they'll give you some homework to do, and do I ever do it? No. (July 2015)

Being isolated in a hut for eight days surely has its benefits in terms of "doing one's homework" and really thinking hard on the therapeutic process at hand. Yet the component of "working with the plants" is fundamental for facilitating the therapeutic encounter, both with ayahuasca and the psychotherapist. Another Takiwasi client, this one from Switzerland, expressed her feelings on the dynamic between the plant diets and ayahuasca:

> I wouldn't say that ayahuasca is the only, the main thing. It really feels to me as if I'm being taken care of maybe a team of doctors and ayahuasca is one of them, and perhaps has an important role in this team. But it really feels like I'm getting assistance from a team. (July 2015)

In this context, the informant is referring to the combinations of plants, ayahuasca, and a therapist as part of one therapeutic team. She had been in the Amazon for a year conducting research, and exemplified that the process of cultural exchange goes both ways as she continued to talk about her conception of the plants as agents that actively aid in the therapeutic process.

> I think when I arrived for the first time here I didn't have any concept at all. I just came without any preconceptions, really open to see what's happening here [at Takiwasi], and then that got fed by my own experiences, plus my interactions with patients and everything. And I think that kind of opened me to the possibilities of what these people were claiming, what the indigenous or native people were saying that the plants are living entities not just in the sense of having a plant body that grows, but maybe on the soul level or on the spirit level that they have. (July 2015)

The flows of knowledge from Amazonian cosmology often become part of the self-narrative of people who partake in ceremonies and plant diets, in a process that Bia Labate (2014) has referred to as a sort of reverse-colonization. Part of this narrative is the local motif of the kind of "work" people are doing when they drink ayahuasca or diet with plants. The notion of work here is a kind of self-work that one does with the plants in order to learn and grow. Plant work is labor toward a new kind of self that is spiritual, healthy, holistic, in touch with nature, and a new cosmology different from that of Western, individualistic thinking. Among traveling foreigners, this work is often done with the image of a more productive, healthier self; an alternative-being that resonates with what Michel Foucault (1988) calls a "technology of the self." Foucault identified four major types of "technologies," of which technologies of the self "permit individuals to effect by their own means or with the help of others a certain number of operations on their own bodies and souls, thoughts, conduct, and way of being, so as to transform themselves in order to attain a certain state of happiness, purity, wisdom, perfection, or immortality" (Foucault 1988, 18). Yet Foucault is clear that technologies of the self do not operate separately from technologies of production, of sign systems, and power. As for the shaman, the work they do is not just on themselves, but also on their clientele and their community.[5] As foreigners become more involved in the cosmology of Peruvian shamanism, the kind of labor in their self-narrative also changes to the extent that they find themselves working through the traumas of their family or ancestors during ceremonies. A young woman who came to diet at Takiwasi spoke of this kind of experience in terms of her mixed Australian and Torres Strait Islander ancestry:

> [I]n ceremonies I hear a lot of messages from my ancestors, yeah, my indigenous ancestors, because essentially through the work that I do in ceremonies and with S*** I'm hoping to heal the traumas, the past traumas through my ancestral lines as well, so they're kind of, I hear them strongly guiding me through the work. (July 2015)

Similarly, a curandero and retreat center owner in Tarapoto told the story of a client who carried the weight of all her emotional experiences in her back (*ella tuvo una experiencia con ayahuacsa fuerte porque ella sentía todo el peso llevaba solo en su espalda*). For this reason, he explained, she was practically crippled with the burden of guilt she felt for her late father, to the extent that she could barely walk, had to wear a girdle, and was dependent on many medications. After eight days of doing a plant diet, she began to walk little by little without assistance, live without the girdle, and emotionally became like a new person. Almost every illness has a psychosomatic origin (*casí todas enfermedes tienen un origen sicosomático*), he concluded: this client needed to rid herself of the oppressive guilt she felt toward her father in order to heal physically. The work with ayahuasca and the diet plants helped her to work through her psychosomatic illness, which related to an intergenerational issue that left her nearly physically crippled.

This sentiment is often repeated in various renditions among both shamans and clientele. The conviction is that people who drink ayahuasca and diet with the plants are enacting a therapeutic process not just for themselves or their immediate clients, but for their ancestral line, their community, or for the previous (often indigenous) inhabitants of the land on which the ceremony is taking place. Thus, this technology of healing is not located just in individual bodies but comes to represent the interconnectedness of selves through both time and space.

CONCLUSION

In a review of recent trends in research on shamanism, Thomas Dubois (2011, 106) states that "More so than virtually any other aspect of contemporary shamanism, the study of entheogens [psychedelics] ties shamanic traditions closely to wider discussion of community-state relations, globalization, and economic networks." This is particularly true for ayahuasca shamanism in the Peruvian Amazon, where global networks of therapists, clients, shamans, NGOs, and tourism companies all contribute to the discourse of a medically plural landscape. In the context of ayahuasca shamanism, as Dubois's comment infers, this landscape is not localized to Peru, but represents a transnational flow of ideas, objects, and people in the form of therapeutic techniques, medicinal plants, practitioners, and clients. To augment the theoretical robustness of the concept of medical pluralism, Hörbst and colleagues propose "medicoscapes," inspired by Appadurai's (1990) focus on following objects and routes of exchange as they pass through different social actors, take on different forms of value, and facilitate interactions often with asymmetrical power dynamics (Hörbst et al. 2017). Medicoscapes embed the concept of medical pluralism within these global flows and social interactions, going beyond the notion of a therapeutic landscape as a bounded cultural or geographic space. This conceptualization is useful for thinking about how ayahuasca shamanism and Western psychology have not only come to coexist as two different epistemologies of healing converging for harm reduction or benefit maximization, but as merging flows of people and technologies that have come to inhabit the same spaces in the Peruvian Amazon.

The concepts of medical pluralism and medical landscapes have been discussed by anthropologists (see Hörbst et al. 2017 for a brief review), yet the concept of therapeutic landscapes is here borrowed from a term first proposed by medical geographer William Gesler (2005) to understand how a place comes to be considered a site of healing and whether a place is authentic in its therapeutic efficacy. Authenticity in this case does not connote how "traditional" a practice is, but how effective a place or practice is in the healing process. In the Peruvian Amazon, and in ayahuasca retreat centers that integrate plant medicine with Western psychotherapy, it is common to hear a traveler say that they did not want to drink ayahuasca in their home country, but felt it was important to come to the jungle and drink with a locally trained shaman, where the plants grow *in situ* and where there is a special energetic power of the forest. The Peruvian Amazon, populated by shamans, forest spirits, rivers, and a growing number of mental health workers, has pivoted from being conceived in the global imagination as a *tierra incognita* full of snakes, jaguars, parasites, and hostile peoples to an authentic site for healing, and where modern populations have a vested interest in increasing the efficacy of its healing power through integrating methods that facilitate the psychological integration of ayahuasca experiences among participants. Several writers argue that in indigenous contexts, the shaman has traditionally functioned as a sort of psychotherapist, and the community as the psycho-integrator for people who undergo strong experiences with sacred plants. However, most modern-day clients do not have this community support, but rather live in societies that stigmatize altered states of consciousness, particularly those induced by psychedelic substances. If the individual suffers because he or she finds it difficult to integrate ayahuasca or plant medicine experiences, they are often blamed for their decisions that caused their own suffering. Instead of a healing process, wider social norms inspire feelings of alienation, sometimes depersonalization, and often a state of confusion as to what the experience meant for their daily lives. As integration therapy continues to develop in both the Amazon and among drinkers of ayahuasca the world over, it remains to be seen whether the reverse colonization of Western styles of thinking persists in altering how Western-trained minds conceive of health and wellness, or whether the asymmetrical relationships between foreign clientele and mental health workers with local practitioners will remain a barrier.

NOTES

1. DMT, or N, N-dimethyltryptamine is short-acting psychedelic from the tryptamine family that is endogenously produced in humans. When ingested orally, its effects are inactivated unless mixed with a monoamine oxidase-A inhibitor. *B. caapi* contains the MAO-inhibitors to permit the oral activation of DMT found in *P. viridis* and *D. cabrerana*, thus the admixture of one of the latter two plants is integral for the effects of ayahuasca. It should also be noted that the names *ayahuasca, chacruna,* and *chaliponga* are just one Quechua-language variation of the names for the plants. Other names for ayahuasca may be indigenous in origin or come from modern neo-religious uses: *datem, yagé, caapi, Nixie Pae, Nishi Cobin, hoasca, daime, la medicina,* and so on.

2. The fieldwork reported was conducted by Olivia Marcus and approved by the University of Connecticut Institutional Review Board. The data presented is part of ongoing fieldwork between 2015 and 2018 among clients, practitioners, and mental health workers associated with shamanic healing centers in San Martín and Loreto.

3. For example: Veterans for Entheogenic Therapy, http://vetentheogenic.squarespace.com/; James Kingsland, "A puke bucket and an ancient drug: is ayahuasca the future of PTSD treatment?" *The Guardian.* April 6, 2017. https://www.theguardian.com/science/blog/2017/apr/06/a-puke-bucket-and-an-ancient-drug-is-ayahuasca-the-future-of-ptsd-treatment-; Andy Coghlan, "Psychedelic drug ayahuasca improves hard-to-treat depression." *New Scientist.* April 14, 2017. https://www.newscientist.com/article/2127802-psychedelic-drug-ayahuasca-improves-hard-to-treat-depression/.

4. In the 1950s, Humphrey Osmond and Abram Hoffer conducted the first studies on psychedelic-assisted psychotherapy with LSD and mescaline, and through the 1970s LSD was used experimentally to treat alcoholics. Similarly, MDMA was used by psychotherapists through the 1970s and early 1980s as a therapeutic adjunct, particularly for the treatment of depression, trauma, and anxiety, until made illegal in 1985 (Sindicich et al. 2010).

5. It is also relevant to note that shamans are constantly working on themselves in order to improve their power as healers and to maintain their own well-being, which involves both warding off spiritual attacks by other shamans and "throwing" attacks at other shamans who threaten themselves, their apprentices, their community, or their clients. Neo-shamans are of course doing similar work on themselves, though rarely embedded in the cosmology of spiritual attacks that is so abundant in the Amazon.

WORKS CITED

Appadurai, Arjun. 1990. "Disjuncture and Difference in the Global Cultural Economy." *Public Culture* 2: 1–24.

Becker, Anne E and Arthur Kleinman. 2013. "Mental health and the global agenda." *New England Journal of Medicine* 369: 66–723.

Becker, Anne, Anjali Motgi, Jonathan Weigel, Giuseppe Raviola, Salmaan Keshavjee, and Arthur Kleinman. 2013. "The unique challenges of mental health and MDRTB." In *Reimagining Global Health*, edited by Paul Farmer, Jim Yong Kim, Arthur Kleinman, and Matthew Basilico, 212–44. University of California Press.

Berlowitz, Ilana, Christian Ghasarian, Heinrich Walt, Fernando Mendive, Vanessa Alvarado, and Chantal Martin-Soelch. 2017. "Conceptions and practices of an integrative treatment for substance use disorders involving Amazonian medicine: traditional healers' perspectives." *Revista Brasileira de Psiquiatra* 40(2): 200–209.

Brabec de Mori, Bernd. 2014. "From the native's point of view: how Shipibo-Konibo experience and interpret ayahuasca drinking with 'gringos.'" In *Ayahuasca Shamanism in the Amazon and Beyond*, edited by Beatriz Caiuby Labate and Clancy Cavnar, 206–30. Oxford University Press.

Bussman, Rainier. 2013. "The Globalization of Traditional Medicine in Northern Peru: From Shamanism to Molecules." *Evidence-Based Complementary and Alternative Medicine: eCAM* DOI:10.1155/2013/291903.

Cohen, Ido. 2017. "Re-turning to wholeness: the psycho-spiritual integration process of ayahuasca ceremonies in western participants from a Jungian perspective." PhD diss., California Institute of Integral Studies, San Francisco.

Constantine, Madonna G, Linda James Myers, Mai Kindaichi, and James L. Moore III. 2004. "Exploring indigenous mental health practices: the roles of healers and helpers in promoting well-being in people of color." *Counseling and Values* 48: 110–25.

Dobkin de Rios, Marlene. 1972. *Visionary Vine: Psychedelic Healing in the Peruvian Amazon*. Prospect Heights, Illinois: Waveland Press.

Dobkin de Rios, Marlene. 1994. Dobkin de Rios. M. 1994. "Drug tourism in the Amazon." *Anthropology of Consciousness* 5(1): 16–19.

DuBois, Thomas A. 2011. "Trends in contemporary research on shamanism." *Numen* 58: 100–128.

Fausto, Carlos. 2004. "A Blend of Blood and Tobacco: Shamans and Jaguars Among the Parakan of Eastern Amazonia." In *In Darkness and Secrecy: The Anthropology of Assault Sorcery and Witchcraft in Amazonia*, edited by Neil L. Whitehead and Robin Wright, 157–78. Durham, NC: Duke University Press.

Fotiou, Evgenia. 2010. "From Medicine Men to Day Trippers: Shamanic Tourism in Iquitos, Peru." PhD diss., University of Wisconsin–Madison.

———. 2014. "On the Uneasiness of Tourism: Considerations on Shamanic Tourism in Western Amazonia." In *Ayahuasca Shamanism in the Amazon and Beyond*, edited by Beatriz Caiuby Labate and Clancy Cavnar, 159–81. Oxford Ritual Studies. New York: Oxford University Press.

———. 2016. "The Globalization of Ayahuasca Shamanism and the Erasure of Indigenous Shamanism." *Anthropology of Consciousness* 27(2): 151–79.

Foucault, Michel. 1988. "Technologies of the Self." In *Technologies of the Self: a seminar with Michel Foucault*, edited by Luther H. Martin, Huck Gutman, and Patrick H. Hutton, 16–49. Amherst: University of Massachusetts Press.

Giove, Rosa. 2012. "Creencias populares sobre la salud mental en Tarapoto." In *Medicinas Tradicionales, Interculturidad y Salud Mental: Memorias del Congreso*

Internacional, Tarapoto 2009, edited by Renaud D'Abaddie, Christine Mikaelian, Patrick Díaz, and Jacques Mabit, 285–93. © Takiwasi Centro de Rehabilitación de Toxicómanos y de Investigación.

González, Débora, María Carvalho, Jordi Cantillo, Aixalá Marc, and Magí Farré. 2017. "Potential Use of Ayahuasca in Grief Therapy." *OMEGA- Journal of Death and Dying*. doi:10.1177/0030222817710879.

Grob, Charles S.1994. "Psychiatric Research with Hallucinogens: What have We Learned?" In *Yearbook of Ethnomedicine*, edited by Christian Ratsch and John R. Baker, 91–112. Berlin: Verlagfyr Wissenschaft und Bildung (VWB).

Grof, Stanislov and Grof, Christina. 1989. *Spiritual Emergency: When Transformation Becomes a Crisis*. New York: Tarcher.

Homan, Joshua. 2017. "Disentangling the ayahuasca boom: local impacts in Western Peruvian Amazonia." In *World Ayahuasca Diaspora*, edited by Beatriz Caiuby Labate, Clancy Cavnar, and Alexander K Gearin, 165–82. London: Routledge.

Horák, Miroslav. 2014. "Comparative Research of Drug Addiction Treatment by the Traditional Indigenous Medicine of Peruvian Amazon and the Matrix® Model." Human and Social Sciences at the Common Conference, November 17–21.

Hörbst Viola, Gerrets Rene, and Pino Schirripa. 2017. "Revisiting medical pluralism." *L'Uomo* 1: 7–26.

Insel, Tom. 2013. Assessing the State of America's Mental Health System. U.S. Department of Health and Human Services, Jan 24, 2013. https://www.nih.gov/sites/default/files/institutes/olpa/20130124-senate-testimony-insel.pdf.

Kakar S. 1982. *Shamans, Mystics, and Doctors*. The University of Chicago Press.

Kiev A. 1968. *Curanderismo: Mexican-American folk psychiatry*. New York: The Free Press.

Labate, Beatriz Caiuby. 2014. "The internationalization of Peruvian vegetalismo." In *Ayahuasca Shamanism in the Amazon and Beyond*, edited by Beatriz Caiuby Labate & Clancy Cavnar, 182–205. Oxford University Press.

Lafrance, Adele, Anja Loizaga-Velder, Jenna Fletcher, Marika Renelli, Natasha Files, and Kenneth W. Tupper. 2017. "Nourishing the Spirit: Exploratory Research on Ayahuasca Experiences along the Continuum of Recovery from Eating Disorders." *Journal of Psychoactive Drugs* 49(5): 427–35.

Lévi-Strauss C. 1963. *Structural Anthropology*. New York: Basic Books, Inc.

Lewis-Fernández, R and Arthur Kleinman. 1994. "Culture, personality, and psychopathology." *Journal of Abnormal Psychology* 103: 67–71.

Mabit, Jacques. 2007. "Ayahuasca in the treatment of Addictions." In *Psychedelic Medicine* (vol. 2), edited by Thomas B. Roberts and Michael J. Winkelmen. Praeger Perspectives.

Mabit, Jacques, Rosa Giove, Joaquín Vega. 1996. "Takiwasi: the use of Amazonian shamanism to rehabilitate drug addicts." In *Yearbook of Cross-Cultural Medicine and Psychotherapy*, edited by Walter Andritzky, 257–85. Berlin, Deutschland: International Institute of Cross-Cultural Therapy Research (IIKT), VWB.

Mabit, Jacques and Claire Sieber. 2006. "The evolution of an experimental drug treatment program using ayahuasca." *Shaman's Drum* 73: 23–31.

Nielson, Jessica L and Julie Megler. 2012. "Consideration of Ayahuasca for the Treatment of Posttraumatic Stress Disorder." *MAPS Bulletin Annual Report*. http://www.maps.org/news-letters/v22n3/v22n3_29-31.pdf.

Noll, Richard. 1983. "Shamanism and schizophrenia: state-specific approach to the 'schizophrenia metaphor' of shamanic states." *American Ethnologist* 10(3): 443–59.

Osório, Flávia L, Rafael F. Sanches, Ligia R. Macedo, Rafael dos Santos, João P. Maia-de-Oliveria, Lauro Wichert-Ana, Draulio B. Araujo, Jordi Riba, José A. Crippa, and Jaime E. Hallak. 2015. "Antidepressant effects of a single dose of ayahuasca in patients with recurrent depression: A preliminary report." *Revista Brasileira de Psiquiatria*, 37(1): 13–20.

Ray, Raven, and Kerry Lassiter. 2016. "Ayahuasca Treatment Center Safety for the Western Seeker." *Anthropology of Consciousness* 27(2): 121–50.

Sanches, Rafael F., Flávia L. Osório, Rafael G. Santos, Ligia R. Macedo, João P. Maia-de-Oliveira, Laura Wichert-Ana, Draulio de Araujo, Jordi Riba, José Crippa, Jaime E. Hallak. 2016. "Antidepressant Effects of a Single Dose of Ayahuasca in Patients with Recurrent Depression: A SPECT Study." *Journal of Clinical Psychopharmacology* 36(1): 77–81.

Santos, Rafael G., Flávia L. Osório, José Alexandre S. Crippa, Jordi Riba, Antônio W. Zuardi, and Jaime E.C. Hallak. 2016. "Antidepressive and anxiolytic effects of ayahuasca: a systematic literature review of animal and human studies." *Revista Brasileira de Psiquiatria* 38(1): 65–72.

Sanz-Biset, Jaime and Salvador Cañigueral. 2011. "Plant use in the medicinal practices known as 'strict diets' in Chazuta valley (Peruvian Amazon)." *Journal of Ethnopharmacology* 137: 271–88.

Saurez-Álvarez, Carlos. 2017. "El paciente siempre tiene la razón." Paper presented at the V Congreso de la Asociación Latinoamericana de Antropología—XVI Congreso de Antropología en Bogotá, Colombia, 6–9 de junio de 2017. https://neip.info/novo/wp-content/uploads/2017/06/Sua percentCC percent81rez_Curanderismo_Amazonico_Occidente_ALA_2017.pdf.

Schmid, Janine T., Henrik Jungaberle, and Rolf Verres. 2010. "Subjective theories about (self-) treatment with ayahuasca." *Anthropology of Consciousness* 21(2): 188–204.

Shanon, Benny. 2002. *The antipodes of the mind: charting the phenomenology of the Ayahuasca experience*. Oxford: Oxford University Press.

Sindicich, Natasha, Louisa Degenhardt, and Wayne Hall. 2010. "The use of MDMA for therapeutic purposes." In *The Health and Psychological Effects of "Ecstasy" (MDMA) Use*, edited by L. Degenhardt and W. Hall. NDARC Monograph #62. Sydney: National Drug and Alcohol Research Centre, University of New South Wales.

Theidon, Kimberly. 2012. *Intimate enemies*. University of Pennsylvania Press.

Thomas, Gerald, Phillipe Lucas, N. Rielle Capler, Kenneth Tupper, and Gina Martin. 2013. "Ayahuasca-Assisted Therapy for Addiction: Results from a Preliminary Observational Study in Canada." *Current Drug Abuse Reviews* 6(1): 30–42.

Torres Romero, Jaime. 2012. "Purgahuasca: aportaciones de la cultura Awajún en el tratamiento de las adicciones." In *Medicinas Tradicionales, Interculturidad y*

Salud Mental: Memorias del Congreso Internacional, Tarapoto 2009, 125–130. © Takiwasi Centro de Rehabilitación de Toxicómanos y de Investigación.

Tupper, Kenneth W. 2008. "The globalization of ayahuasca: Harm reduction or benefit maximization?" *International Journal of Drug Policy* 19: 297–303.

Vigo, Daniel, Graham Thorncroft, and Rifat Atun. 2016. "Estimating the true global burden of mental illness." *The Lancet Psychiatry* 3(2): 171–78.

Vitebsky, Piers. 2003. "From Cosmology to Environmentalism: Shamanism as Local Knowledge in a Global Setting." In *Shamanism: A Reader*, edited by Graham Harvey, 276–98. London: Routledge.

Vollenweider, Franz, and Michael Kometer. 2010. "The neurobiology of psychedelic drugs: implications for the treatment of mood disorders." *Nature Reviews Neuroscience*, 11(9): 642–51.

Chapter Seven

Queer Families in the Margins

Considering Gender and Health in U.S.-Andean Gay Adoptions

Ronnie Anthony Shepard
and Shir Lerman Ginzburg

While Colombia has historically been one of the most progressive countries in South America regarding the rights of the LGBTQ population (homosexual acts were decriminalized in 1980), in March 2011, equality was far from guaranteed. At the time, Chandler Burr, curator of the Museum of Art and Design in New York City, had just completed the two-year process of legally adopting his sons from the country. Burr, who self-identifies as gay, kept his sexuality private throughout the adoption process, and the brothers, a "special needs" and "hard-to-place" sibling-set due to their age (ten and six at the time) and familial relationship, were released into his care. As the new family prepared to leave for their home in the United States, Burr let slip to an official from Colombia's Family Welfare Institute (ICBF) that the situation was terrible for people like himself who wanted to adopt children in Colombia but could not, due to their sexual orientation. The news did not go over well, with the official blocking Burr from taking the boys, his legally recognized sons, out of the country. With his casual revelation, a prominent court case began as one man fought for the right to adopt despite his sexuality (El Tiempo 2012).[1]

This chapter endeavors to map the gendered nature of same-sex international adoptions between the United States and the Andean Community.[2] While adoption is normally described as simply "a form of filiation (creating parent-child links)" (Bowie 2004, 5), this basic definition neglects the surge of gay singles and couples contemplating familial expansion across international borders, and has made consideration of current adoption trends particularly salient. Quite simply, adoption is a gendered process which is negotiated at multiple levels simultaneously: international, economic, cultural, social, and familial. Using the Burr case as a jumping off point, we begin with a discussion of the cross-cultural adoption issues facing both LGBTQ potential parents and the children in need of homes. From this point, we move into an examination of the gendered nature of adoption within and from the Andean Community, noting that while in many cases it is possible for single parents to adopt, in some cases the process is much easier for females than males (and even married couples), and it is almost always at the expense of hiding their sexuality, same-sex relationships, and/or potential co-parents. Currently, Colombia has its own unique restrictions, and is now the only Andean country in which sexuality is not a primary determinant in the international adoption process, largely due to the Burr case.

There are exceptions to every rule, however, and the adoption process is no exception. In this case, the primary exception is the health and perceived "special needs" of the children made available for adoption. We discuss several of the often-minor issues faced by the children, noting the changes that may take a child from the role of "healthy child," to one considered "hard to place." Finally, we consider several actions that can be taken to help LGBTQ parents with the adoption process, with the goal of giving children the families they deserve and moving queer families out of the margins.

CROSS-CULTURAL ADOPTION ISSUES

During the course of Burr's fight to regain custody of his adopted children, the boys expressed their desire to remain with their father, proving a certain malleability exists between parents and children in cross-cultural adoptions. For example, in Kosack's temporary adoption of a native Cameroonian child she asked herself whether it was legitimate to take a child from the culture in which it was born and place it into another, even if the child's life chances were significantly improved, and whether this seismic cultural shift would provoke a conflict of identity in the adopted child (Kosack 2004). It stands to reason that removing a child from its native culture and placing it into both a new culture and a home with same-sex parents would initially be even more jarring. However, these changes should not necessarily be seen as a negative. In Burr's case, the children wanted to be with their father, and all of the other issues surrounding the case were insignificant when compared to the bond created between them. The children simply moved from an outsider status in their country of birth due to their lack of a familial unit, to a liminal outsider status in their new home due to the newfound familial structure and Latin American-to-North American cultural differences.

In some international adoption cases, "adoption agencies may perpetuate the 'myth of the orphan' and present their services as a solution to Third World poverty, and adoptive parents, through ignorance or a willingness to collude, may fail to ask sufficiently searching questions concerning the adoption process" (Bowie 2004, 14). In Burr's case, however, the media's depiction was not presented as a case of the "First World savior rescuing the children from the shackles of Third World poverty," but as a man and two children attempting to reunite after the familial bond had already been formed.

Just as there are myriad reasons prospective parents may choose to adopt a child, there are many reasons why biological parents may choose to place a child for adoption. Within Latin American adoptions, economic survival can be considered a chief mitigating factor. In these cases, we find that children capable of contributing income may be assigned from one household to another in either a fostering situation, a formalized adoption, or through a hybridization of the two. Secondly, labor must be balanced by age and gender, facilitating the movement of children between families and homes. Here, we find that women in households with an excess of men and a shortage of female support may be susceptible to an illness colloquially known as *debilidad*. Women in these cases are responsible for meeting the productive demands associated with the female role in a patriarchal society, as well as providing the domestic services related to the care of large numbers of males. Finally, there is a strong desire to have children of both sexes in the home. This desire reflects the interests of both men and women in collecting "assistants" of their own gender (Anderson 2009). In all these cases, a heteronormative home life with a strict house/street divide—the norm in a patriarchal system—is considered ideal, leaving one to wonder where prospective LGBTQ parents and potential adoptive LGBTQ children fit in.

As noted by Bowie, "in Western societies the term 'adoption' is conventionally used for the transference of full parental rights from birth to social parents, in contrast to fostering, in which only a partial transfer occurs" (Bowie 2004, 5). Transitioning from fostering a domestic child to adopting said child is by far the most economically advantageous to prospective parents both gay and straight, and protects both the parents and the children from the prejudices and legal issues found in cross-cultural intercountry adoptions.

LEGALITIES OF GENDERED ADOPTIONS IN THE ANDEAN COMMUNITY

In Colombia, the case of Chandler Burr and his children was considered a done deal. All the requisite fees inherent to the adoption process had been paid, and the waiting periods had been completed at the time of the incident. The adoption of the children had gone through all the proper channels. The family's bond had been confirmed by outside officials and the adoption was

Table 7.1. Andean Adoption Restrictions based on Gender and Heterosexual Marital Status[1]

	Single males	*Single females*	*Married couples*
Bolivia boys	Birth +	Birth +	Birth +
Bolivia girls	Birth +	Birth +	Birth +
Bolivia additional restrictions:	U.S. citizens must be legal residents of Bolivia to adopt from Bolivia. Both single and married applicants are welcome. Potential parents must be 25–50 years of age or 15 years older than the adopted child.		
Colombia boys	8+	8+	Birth +
Colombia girls	–	8+	Birth +
Colombia additional restrictions:	Couples should be married a minimum of one year. Potential parents should be 25–50 years of age. No more than one divorce per applicant. No more than 45 years between the parent and the child they wish to adopt.		
Ecuador boys	8+	–	Birth +
Ecuador girls	–	5+	Birth +

Ecuador additional restrictions:	Both members of a married couple must be at least 25 years old and married for at least 3 years. There must be at least a 14-year age difference between the child and the youngest parent.		
	Married couples must be heterosexual.		
Peru boys	5+	5+	Birth +
Peru girls	5+	5+	Birth +
Peru additional restrictions:	Married parents aged 25–43 qualify to adopt a child up to age 3. Married parents aged 44–50 qualify to adopt a child 3–6 years old. Married parents aged 51–55 qualify to adopt a child aged 6 and up. Potential single parents aged 35–50 may adopt a child age 5 and up. Prospective parents must be at least 18 years older than the child. Inter-country adoptions are restricted to children deemed legally abandoned.		

[1]All current intercountry adoption restrictions can be found at the U.S. Department of State—Bureau of Consular Affairs website: https://travel.state.gov/content/travel/en/Intercountry-Adoption/Intercountry-Adoption-Country-Information.html.

approved, until the one moment in which he mentioned his sexuality. For his part, Burr acknowledged keeping his sexuality a secret during the entirety of the adoption process, saying: "I'm not stupid. I know that in Colombia, as in other places in the world, there are people that have prejudices." In this case, the official's internalized prejudices intersected with structural adoption restrictions to create a years-long waiting period in which the ones who lost the most were the children.

As seen in table 7.1, restrictions on the adoption process vary considerably among Andean nations based on gender, age, and marital status. Except in the case of Colombia, where single females are allowed to adopt children of both sexes, neither gender has a greater access to children based solely on sex characteristics. Restrictions are not only placed on the prospective parents, but on the children, as well. In Ecuador, children can only be adopted if they are abandoned, if birth parents have consented to give up parental responsibilities, and other near relatives relinquish their care-giving role (Leifsen 2004, 190). The legalities become even more complex when we consider that many of the children do not live with their birth parents but in institutions where the possibility of being caught in legal limbo is relatively high (Leifsen 2004, 189). It is worth noting that while the sexuality of the potential parents is almost always a deterrent to the adoption process, there are no current restrictions based on the sexual identities of the children.

As Leifsen notes in his discussion of Ecuadorian children and international adoption, "the situation is totally different in the USA where numerous private adoption agencies and adoption lawyers offer their services, which in principle are open to any applicant regardless of place of origin. Hence, the variation in types of adoption agencies is considerable and applicants have an opportunity to make a choice that matches their values and expectations" (Leifsen 2004, 188). These agencies often vary significantly in funding and infrastructure, and the burden of sustaining the orphanages is passed on to the potential parents through fees and involuntary "donations." Duncan (2000) recognizes that intercountry adoptions are not solely about family building, as they have also become sources of income.

In table 7.2, we can see that intercountry adoptions between the Andean Community and the United States can be a cost-prohibitive process for even the most dedicated and/or deserving of potential parents. Bolivia, with the most economical range of costs on the scale, can attribute its "reasonable" rates to the fact that potential parents are required to be legal Bolivian residents as opposed to travelers from abroad. Yet, when it comes to the economic realities of adoption, the parents (both biological and adoptive) have no say in the valuation of the child. Says Leifsen:

Table 7.2. Estimated Costs of Single-Child Andean-U.S. International Adoptions by Country[3]

Country	*Estimated Cost of Adoption*
Bolivia	\$5,000–\$7,000
Colombia	\$12,000–\$30,000
Ecuador	\$25,000–\$40,000
Peru	~\$26,000

Most recent costs for adoption can be found at the websites of those individual U.S.-based adoption agencies that cater to transnational adoptions from Andean nations, or from clearinghouse-style websites such as www.adopt.com and www.adoption.com.

> The adoptive parents, for example, can stress the emotional dimensions concerning the adoption, but they cannot significantly annul the money transaction involved or influence the size of the adoption fee. Similarly, the birthparents cannot control the ways their child is connected to formal and informal payments from the moment they give up the baby. Neither can the adoption agencies eliminate irregular economic activity in relation to the adoption process (2004, 183).

While the monetization of children and families can be an off-putting proposition for many, as noted by Selman, "there are still many children in institutions in poor countries, especially those with special needs, who desperately need a family and, for some of these, intercountry adoptions can offer new hope" (Selman 2004, 270). Yet, the definition of "special needs" is bound in time and space, shifting to coincide with the wants of the adoption facilitators and the needs of the children waiting for families of their own.

UNDERSTANDING THE "SPECIAL NEEDS" OF ADOPTION

Defining Special Needs

Adopting a child with special needs is an intricate process, partly due to the complexity of defining "special needs." The 1993 Hague Adoption Convention, which monitors international adoptions between the United States and the other Convention signatories, has several guidelines to ensure child health and safety, including growing up in a positive family environment and the prevention of child abductions and trafficking (Hague Convention 1993). However, the Convention does not define special needs, but rather leaves this definition to each signatory nation. The United States federal government does not have a federal definition of special needs, but rather allows individual states to determine the definition. Factors that influence the determination of special needs includes age, medical, physical, or emotional disabilities, risk of such disabilities based on birth family, and any condition that makes placing a child with an adoptive family more difficult. All states except Georgia, Idaho, Minnesota, and Pennsylvania state that a non-Hispanic white child above a certain age (generally eight or nine) is deemed to have special needs.[4] All states indicate that a child of a minority group (e.g., African American, Hispanic) is considered to have special needs if adopted after the age of two or three. The U.S. government also does not have specific legal requirements to determine eligibility for families who wish to adopt children with special needs; the federal government leaves this decision to the individual states. According to Title IV-E of the Social Security Act, in order for a child to be eligible for federal adoption assistance, a child with special needs must meet the following two requirements in addition to meeting state requirements: the child should not or cannot be returned to his or her birth parent(s), and an unsuccessful attempt should already have been made to find a home for the child without the assistance of an adoption agency (except where such a placement would have placed the child at a disadvantage).

Ecuador, Colombia, and Peru are Convention signatories, and have similar guidelines to those in the United States for defining a child as having special needs and for prospective parent eligibility (U.S. Department of State 2014). Neither country has a specific definition for special needs per se but define "disability" based on the World Health Organization's guidelines. Colombia's Disability Act uses the word "limitations" instead of "disability," and these are defined as a temporary or permanent physical, mental, or sensory impairment that impedes an individual's ability to perform daily activities and is aggravated by social and/or economic environments. Single parents over twenty-five can adopt children seven or older on a case-by-case basis, and common-law spouses are permitted to adopt, as well (U.S. Department of State 2014a). Ecuador's Chapter II of Executive Decree 3603 defines a person with a disability as someone whose ability to perform an activity within a normal range is reduced by at least 30 percent, preventing that individual from performing daily activities. Single parents can only adopt children of the same sex, and the parent must be at least fourteen years older than the child. If the prospective parents are married, they must be in a heterosexual relationship (U.S. Department of State 2014b). In Peru, single parents between 35 and 50 can adopt children five years and older; Peru only allows heterosexual couples to adopt, and single gay, lesbian, bisexual, transgender, and intersex individuals may be unable to adopt children (U.S. Department of State 2014c). Peru's Law 27050, the "General Law of the Person with Disability," defines disability as the significant physical, mental, or sensorial loss of function that prevents an individual from conducting normal activity (Mental Disability Rights International 2004).

Children with special needs are considered the top priority in adoption cases in both the United States and in the Andes. Children living in socially undesirable conditions make up a significant portion of special-needs cases (Hegar and Watson 2013; Leinaweaver and Seligmann 2009; Rosenthal 1993). Socially undesirable factors include, but are not limited to, older age, poverty, sexual or physical violence, HIV and AIDS, mental illnesses, and behavioral problems (Jones 2012; Leinaweaver and Seligmann 2009; Rosenthal 1993; Somma et al. 2008). White married couples in higher socioeconomic status groups are more highly preferred as adoptive parents in the unspoken adoption hierarchy, and as a result, LGBTQ couples, non-white couples, and single parents are given children with special needs, who are themselves generally less preferred (NAIC 2014). As a result, children in orphanages and foster care are disproportionately of African and Hispanic descent (McKenzie 1993). Coupled with a decrease in the availability of healthy children and an increase in children with special needs (van Wichelen 2014), the competitiveness for socially desirable children has increased, contributing to an ethical dilemma in which the medicalization of international child adoptions and the entangled legalities of international politics constitute the playing field for social inequality and the preference for the social status quo. With same-sex marriage a controversial topic in many parts of the world, international politics concerning who is an acceptable parent are negotiated, with the state acting as a surrogate paternalistic figure until the authorities find prospective parents that they deem appropriate. Bolivia and Ecuador do not permit same-sex couples to adopt children while Peru only permits heterosexual married couples to adopt (Wardle 2013), and Russia has prohibited couples from countries permitting same-sex marriages—Colombia is one of a handful of South American countries with legalized same-sex marriages—to adopt Russian children, regardless of the prospective parents' sexual orientation (Sonne 2014). However, with fewer healthy children available for adoption, there is a dire need for parents to adopt children with special needs, and single parents are sought to adopt the children left behind.

Adoption agencies try to have birth siblings adopted together whenever possible, although this proves to be more difficult when the prospective parents already have birth children (Rosenthal 1993). Research suggests that children that are adopted into different households from their birth siblings show higher rates of emotional and behavioral problems (Groza et al. 2003). It is beneficial for children with other special needs to be placed into the same household as their siblings, as the siblings can offer emotional support, and the household can offer more personalized attention for the child with special needs than if the child were in a household with other children with special needs (AdoptUSKids 2014).

Determinants of Special Needs

Poverty is one of the single biggest contributors to illness worldwide (Dettrick et al. 2013; Hadley and Crooks 2012; Jackson et al. 2009; López-Cevallos and Chi 2012b). Three out of four people in the Andes live below the poverty lines of their respective countries, and the region has the poorest populations in South America (International Fund for Agricultural Development 2014). Indigenous communities and single-parent households are the most vulnerable to poverty in the Andes (López-Cevallos and Chi 2012a). Poverty is also a contributing factor in the development of mental and physical special needs and adoptions (Christoffersen 2012; Waldman et al. 2010). Families that cannot financially support a child may put that child up for adoption, and this is particularly true if the child has a physical or mental disability that requires medical care that is above and beyond what the family can afford (Hegar and Watson 2013). Caring for sick children places incredible strain on the parents (especially mothers), making the parents more prone to getting sick themselves and impeding the development of the parent-child relationship (Roy 2011). Parents in poor families are also more likely to lack basic work standards, such as health care for themselves or dependents, sick leave, or time off to care for a sick child (Dettrick et al. 2013; López-Cevallos and Chi 2012a; McGibbon 2012). In Ecuador, staggering economic differences contribute to unequal access to health care, with a third of the population unable to afford regular health care (López-Cevallos and Chi 2009; López-Cevallos and Chi 2012b).

Parents of low socioeconomic status may not be able to afford the health care to care for both themselves and their children and may give their children up for adoption in the hope that their children will have better options elsewhere (McGibbon 2012; Waldman et al. 2010). This concept is known in Peru as *superar* ("improving oneself"), namely overcoming poverty through self-improvement (Leinaweaver 2008a). This is especially true for children with special needs, whose parents will circulate them to other families so that their children may have better health care and improved chances for overall survival and success. The aim of *superar*, and the general Andean practice of circulating non-related children, can be connected to the concept of *ayllu*, or the traditional Quechua and Aymara concept of community (Leinaweaver 2008b; Newberry 2009). An *ayllu* is a government-protected system of extended family networks, and the networks include the adoption of non-related individuals. Children in this system could be circulated within the kin network to members that can better provide for the children, especially if the children in question have special needs and require more attention and care.

Since the 1990s, a growing number of adoptions in developed countries are children that come from developing and under-developed countries (Leinaweaver and Seligmann 2009), so acknowledging the adoption of children from such countries is essential. Children with disabilities are much more likely to experience forms of material hardship (e.g., food insecurity, no income or health insurance) than people without disabilities, even after controlling for income and other characteristics (McGibbon 2012; Waldman et al. 2010). Children who are poor have little chance of overcoming the disadvantages associated with poverty; poverty during childhood has a range of lasting detrimental effects, and children with preexisting health problems have decreased chances of surviving the additional health problems that are associated with poverty (Budrys 2010).

HIV and AIDS status are common reasons for putting a child up for adoption in the Andes (Fernandez et al. 2005; Salazar et al. 2009). While the epidemic in the region is concentrated primarily among men who have sex with men (Salazar et al. 2009), it is also found in children. Adoptions of children with HIV and AIDS are becoming increasingly common, particularly as the health care for children with HIV and AIDS is better in the United States, and people with HIV are protected from discrimination under the Americans with Disabilities Act. HIV is transmitted prenatally as well as sexually, and mothers with HIV may not be able to financially or emotionally care for a child with HIV if they themselves need to cope with the illness. Already struggling with anxiety about the stigma associated with HIV, mothers may put their children up for adoption to either mitigate their own anxiety or to try and provide their children with a better future (Campbell and Gibbs 2009). Many countries in Latin America, including those in the Andes, also do not have sufficient or well-maintained programs to help people with HIV. This is due at least partly to declining economies and to starkly unequal economic distributions between socioeconomic groups, leading to a lack of sufficient medication for the entire population (Fernandez et al. 2005; Stillwaggon 2000). In much of the region, HIV is associated with homosexuality, which is likewise stigmatized, leading to heterosexual men rejecting their HIV status, denying having infected their children via the mothers, and disowning children with HIV (Fernandez et al. 2005). Due to the perceived association between HIV and homosexuality, children that come out as gay may also be considered undesirable regardless of their actual HIV status, and subsequently disowned. The estimate for people of all ages living with HIV in Ecuador in 2008 was 26,000 (IFRC 2008); as of 2011, there were thirty children born with HIV in Ecuador (UNAIDS 2012). UNAIDS estimated in 2001 that roughly 4,000 children under the age of fifteen were living with HIV and AIDS in Colombia (Watchlist 2004), and by 2007, that number was 230,000, including older teenagers ages fifteen to nineteen (Children of the Andes 2007).

In addition to HIV and AIDS, the adoption of children with other special needs has become more common. For example, international couples are increasingly adopting children with cleft palates (Hansson et al. 2012; Hansson et al. 2013). Children with these special needs are often ostracized in their home countries due to the common perception that they were conceived and born in sin. In Ecuador and Peru, from pre-Colombian contact until at least the Middle Ages, children with cleft palates were thought to have faces similar to hares, and thus to be animal-human hybrids and a shame to their families (Wright 2012). Furthermore, care providers in orphanages are not always prepared to help children with these special needs (Lygnegård et al. 2013), leading to increased developmental delays.

Mental illnesses are prevalent in Latin American countries, and treatment for said illnesses is underfunded and limited in scope (Minnetti et al. 2012). International adoptees are at increased risk for developing depression, anxiety, attention deficit hyperactivity disorder, and conduct disorders (Juffer and van IJzendoorn 2005). The length of time that children live in orphanages and/or foster homes prior to adoption directly contributes to developmental delays and mental illnesses, which contribute to the difficulty in finding adoptive parents for older children (Melås et al. 2014; Minnis et al. 2006; van London et al. 2007). Children often face neglect, psychological deprivation, inadequate health services, and maternal separation while living in orphanages; these factors lead to the increased likelihood of mental illnesses and behavioral problems (Juffer and van IJzendoorn 2005). Additionally, prolonged experience with the foster care system contributes to emotional trauma and increased exposure to violence, alcoholism, and multiple separations from foster families (Desai et al. 2012; McKenzie 1993). Children who are successfully adopted internationally have improved physical and mental development as compared to children living in orphanages and foster homes (Christoffersen 2012; van IJzendoorn et al. 2005). However, the majority of internationally adopted children successfully form stable relationships and develop normally compared to their age groups, especially if adopted at a younger age (van London et al. 2007). There is little hard data on incidence and prevalence rates of mental illnesses in Colombia and Ecuador, particularly among children. However, mental illnesses are directly correlated with violence (Kilpatrick et al. 2003; Van Dorn et al. 2012), and with Colombia's population still suffering from the side effects of prolonged warfare, it can be speculated that mental illnesses are higher in the country than are currently reported. Additionally, high rates of poverty, teen suicide, and domestic violence in Ecuador constitute mental health issues and a profound need for more developed mental health prevention and treatment programs in that country (Cruza-Guet et al. 2009).

Women and children in the Andes experience violence in their homes at a disproportionately high rate compared to men (McGibbon 2012; Van Vleet 2002); this is particularly true for children with special needs (Jones et al. 2012; WHO 2014). Special needs are often individualized and blamed on an individual's genetics, behavior, and lifestyle, rather than on macro-level problems (such as poverty, food insecurity, and domestic violence) that contribute to illness (Birn et al. 2009; McGibbon and Hallstrom 2012). Macro-level factors contribute to developmental delays in utero, leading to physical disabilities, anxiety, depression, and increased traumatic stress later in life (McGibbon 2012), all of which are highly stigmatized illnesses (Brown et al. 2010; Goffman 1963; Link et al. 2008). Children with mental illnesses or behavioral problems are generally over-represented in the adoption system, particularly if they are from low-income families, as their parents do not have the ability and/or desire to care for them (Burns et al. 2004; Oswald et al. 2010; Pasztor et al. 2006). Oftentimes the children are blamed for having a mental illness or behavioral problem. Presently, no significant statistics have been released on the number of children with mental illnesses or behavioral problems in the adoption system in the Andes.

For families and communities that cannot or will not support children with special needs, orphanages and adoptions are often the only option available. There are several options for Americans that wish to adopt children in the Andes with special needs. Lifeline, for example, is a certified adoption agency, and is certified to work in Colombia and Peru, in addition to several countries in Central America and the Caribbean.[5] Lifeline is a Christian adoption agency: it specifies that the potential parents must be married for at least three years prior to the adoption, does not permit single-parent adoptions, and requires that potential parents promise to raise the children as Christians. Bethany Christian Services is another adoption agency and permits the adoption of children with mild to severe special needs. Couples must be married for at least two years prior to the adoption, and the agency does not allow couples with more than one divorce per person to adopt children. Prospective parents that are HIV positive or have a history of cancer or substance abuse are not eligible. Single women (but not single men) can adopt, but they are restricted to children that are at least seven and/or have special needs. Fundamor, an orphanage on the outskirts of Cali, Colombia, is dedicated to helping children with HIV and AIDS. Beginning July 15, 2013, ICBF (the Instituto Colombiano del Bienestar Familiar, or the Colombian Institute for Family Welfare) stopped accepting new inter-country adoption applications from non-Colombian citizens living abroad that were interested in adopting a child under six years and eleven months old (slightly under the age of seven). An exception is made if ICBF considers the child to have special characteristics or needs. The United States government recommends that all gay and lesbian persons wishing to adopt a child from Colombia consult with the ICBF concerning Colombia's legal requirements, prior to initiating the adoption process.

CHANDLER BURR IN CONTEXT

The case of Chandler Burr, the gay New York journalist who tried to adopt two Colombian siblings, fits the definition of international special-needs adoptions. The ICBF approved Mr. Burr's application—Mr. Burr met the two boys and got along with them—before Mr. Burr let slip to an ICBF agent that he was gay. The agent reported the comment, and the ICBF took the two boys back from Mr. Burr. Ultimately, Mr. Burr was allowed to keep the boys due to changes in the penal code signed into effect shortly before his adoption case. The law prohibits discrimination on the basis of sexual orientation. Coincidentally, the two boys are considered to have special needs due both to their ages (thirteen and nine) and to their status as siblings; both factors make it more difficult to place children with parents. However, the boys' special needs were not considered in this case, which was decided solely on the new anti-discrimination law.

FINAL THOUGHTS

In May 2012, for the first time in the history of the country, the Colombian judicial system granted adoption rights to a homosexual man. With the landmark court decision, Chandler Burr was allowed to leave Colombia with his two sons—then aged ten and thirteen—legally adopted at the beginning of 2011. Colombia did not have another adoption case with such significance to the LGBTQ community until August 2014, when, for the first time, the country's constitutional court allowed a native Colombian lesbian couple to adopt a child born to one of its mothers through artificial insemination (Associated Press: 2014). Since then, LGBTQ rights have progressed at a rapid pace, with same-sex adoption rights codified in November 2015, and same-sex marriage legalized in April 2016. As far as the results of the Burr case are concerned, he shares, "Now, we are living on the outskirts of New York and they are attending a good school. My mother supports me in their care." While the happy ending found in this case bodes well for LGBTQ *parents*, it says nothing of the plight of LGBTQ *children*.

During the process of adoption, biological facts are overwritten by social facts (Leifsen 2004). In a recent article chronicling the challenges faced by LGBTQ youth in the United States' foster care system, Colby Swettberg of Massachusetts-based Adoption & Foster Care Mentoring notes the declining interest of LGBTQ parents in fostering gay and lesbian youths as the potential for gay adoptions becomes a reality. In a sobering affirmation, Robin McHaelen, executive director of True Colors, Inc., a non-profit organization dedicated to the needs of LGBTQ youth, notes, "many of our kids have been told they're not family-appropriate: 'We're not even going to look for a family for you. We're going to look for a group home'" (Kennedy 2013). In their quest to find the perfect child, perhaps potential LGBTQ parents should not forget to also look closer to home. In any event, the one thing that can be agreed on is that "there is no single message or right way of doing things, or any simplistic lessons that can be drawn from a cross-cultural approach to adoption" (Bowie 2004: 16). While the steps taken may seem small, they cannot help but move queer families into the mainstream and further away from society's margins.

NOTES

1. All references to this case are taken from an interview between Burr and Colombia's *El Tiempo* newspaper, published on May 24, 2012 and electronically archived at http://www.eltiempo.com/archivo/documento/CMS-11865445.
2. This paper uses the traditional description of the Andean Community as consisting of Bolivia, Colombia, Ecuador, and Peru.
3. While all adoption agencies are able to set their own rates and estimated costs, according to our research, only one agency provides an estimated cost of adoption from Peru accessible to potential parents through internet websites. The U.S. Department of State has no further information, either, leading us to assume that estimated costs will only rise from the $26,000 estimated by adoptive parents at http://stillwewait.wordpress.com/2013/01/21/peru-country-profile/
4. The specified states do not have age requirements for non-Hispanic white children to be determined "special needs."
5. Costa Rica, the Dominican Republic, Haiti, and Honduras.

WORKS CITED

Adopt.com. 2010. "Peru." http://adopt.com/peru/.
Adoption.com. 2014. "Bolivia." http://bolivia.adoption.com/foreign/adopting-from-bolivia-factsheet,3.html.

AdoptUSKids. 2014. "Ten Myths and Realities about Sibling Adoption." http://www.adoptuskids.org/_assets/files/NRCRRFAP/resources/ten-myths-and-realities-of-sibling-adoptions.pdf.

Anderson, Jeanine. 2009. "Assembling and Disassembling Families." *Journal of Latin American and Caribbean Anthropology* 14, no. 1: 185–198.

Associated Press. 2014. "Colombia Allows Lesbian Partner to Adopt Child Born via Artificial Insemination." http://www.lgbtqnation.com/2014/08/colombia-allows-lesbian-partner-to-adopt-child-born-via-artificial-insemination/.

Battiste, Marie, James [Sa'Ke'j] Youngblood Henderson. 2012. "Oppression and the Health of Indigenous Peoples." In *Oppression: A Social Determinant of Health*, edited by E.A. McGibbon, 89–96. Halifax & Winnipeg: Fernwood Publishing.

Bowie, Fiona. 2004. "Adoption and the Circulation of Children: A Comparative Perspective." In *Cross-Cultural Approaches to Adoption*, edited by F. Bowie, 3–20. New York: Routledge.

Building Your Family: The Infertility and Adoption Guide. 2014. "Ecuador Adoption Fast Facts." http://buildingyourfamily.com/adoption/international-adoption-countries/ecuador-adoption/.

Burns, Barbara J., Susan D. Phillips, H. Ryan Wagner, Richard P. Barth, David J. Kolko, Yvonne Campbell, and John Landsver. 2004. "Mental Health Need and Access to Mental Health Services by Youths Involved with Child Welfare: A National Survey." *Journal of the American Academy of Child & Adolescent Psychiatry* 43, no. 8: 960–970.

Campbell, Catherine and Andrew Gibbs. 2009. "Stigma, Gender and HIV: Case Studies of Inter-sectionality." In *Gender and HIV/AIDS: Critical Perspectives from the Developing World*, edited by J. Boesten and Nana K. Poky, 29–46. Burlington, VT: Ashgate Publishing Company.

Children's Home Society of Minnesota. 2013. "Ecuador." http://www.chsfs.org/AdoptFromEcuador.

Christoffersen, Mogens Nygaard. 2012. "A Study of Adopted Children, Their Environment, and Development: A Systematic Review." *Adoption Quarterly* 15, no. 3: 220–237.

Cruza-Guet, María-Cristina, Arnold R. Spokane, Carlos León-Andrade, and Teresa Borja. 2009 "Diversity, Hegemony, Poverty, and the Emergence of Counseling Psychology in Ecuador." In *International Handbook of Cross-Cultural Counseling: Cultural Assumptions and Practices Worldwide*, edited by L.H. Gerstein, Seung-Ming Alvin Leung, and Kathryn L. Norsworthy, 393–402. Thousand Oaks, CA: Sage Publications, Inc.

Desai, Rani A., John Chapman, Paul R. Falzer, and Randy Borum. 2012. "Mental Illness, Violence Risk, and Race in Juvenile Detention: Implications for Disproportionate Minority Contact." *American Journal of Orthopsychiatry* 32, no. 1: 32–40.

Dettrick, Zoe, Sonja Firth, and Eliana Jimenez Soto. 2013. "Do Strategies to Improve Quality of Maternal and Child Health Care in Lower and Middle Income Countries Lead to Improved Outcomes? A Review of the Evidence." *PLoS One* 8, no. 12: 1–9.

Everett, Margaret and Josef N. Wieland. 2013. "Diabetes among Oaxaca's Transnational Population: An Emerging Syndemic." *Annals of Anthropological Practice* 36, no. 2: 295–311.

Fernandez, M. Isabel, Jeffrey A. Kelly, L. Yvonne Stevenson, Cheryl A. Sitzler, Jorge Hurtado, Claudina Valdez, Felipe Vallejo, Anton M. Somlai, Yuri A. Amirkanian, Eric G. Benotsch, Kevin D. Brown, and Karen M. Opgennorth. 2005. "HIV prevention programs of nongovernmental organizations in Latin America and the Caribbean: The Global AIDS Intervention Network project." *Revista Panamericana de Salud Pública* 17, no. 3: 154–162.

Freundlich, Madelyn. 2000. "Adoption and Ethics: The Role of Race, Culture, and National Origin in Adoption," edited by M. Freundlich, vol. 1. Washington, DC: Child Welfare League of America.

Gladney Center for Adoption. 2014. "Colombia." http://adoptionsbygladney.com/adoption/international/colombia-adoption-faq.

Groza, Victor, Connie Maschmeier, Cheryl Jamison, and Trista Piccola. 2003. "Siblings and Out-of-Home Placement: Best Practices." *Families in Society* 84, no. 4: 480–490.

Hague Convention. 1993. "Convention on Protection of Children and Co-operation in Respect of Intercountry Adoption." Hague convention on intercountry adoption, The Hague, The Netherlands, 1993.

Hansson, Emma, Henry Svensson, and Magnus Becker. 2012. "Adopted children with cleft lip or palate, or both, require special needs cleft surgery." *Journal of Plastic Surgery and Hand Surgery* 46, no. 2: 75–79.

Hansson, Emma, Jenny Östman, and Magnus Becker. 2013. "Adopting a child with cleft lip and palate: A study of parents' experiences." *Journal of Plastic Surgery and Hand Surgery* 47, no. 1: 30–35.

Illien Adoptions International, Inc. 2013. "Ecuador Adoption Program." http://www.illienadoptions.org/ecuador_adoption.html.

International Fund for Agricultural Development. 2014. "Rural Poverty in Americas." http://www.ruralpovertyportal.org/region/home/tags/americas.

Jones, Lisa, Mark A. Bellis, Sara Wood, Karen Hughes, Ellie McCoy, Lindsay Eckley, Geoff Bates, Christopher Mikton, Tom Shakespeare, and Alana Officer. 2012. "Prevalence and risk of violence against children with disabilities: a systematic review and meta-analysis of observational studies." *The Lancet* 380, no. 9845: 899–907.

Juffer, Femmie and Marinus H. van IJzendoorn. 2005. "Behavior Problems and Mental Health Referrals of International Adoptees: A Meta-Analysis." *Journal of the American Medical Association* 293, no. 20: 2501–2515.

Kennedy, Kelli. 2013. "Gay Foster Kids' Discrimination Battle Heats Up in States." http://www.huffingtonpost.com/2013/06/22/gay-foster-kids-discrimination-_n_3483473.html?utm_hp_ref=email_share.

Kilpatrick, Dean G., Kenneth J. Ruggiero, Ron Acierno, Benjamin E. Saunders, Heidi S. Resnick, and Connie L. Best. 2003. "Violence and Risk of PTSD, Major Depression, Substance Abuse/Dependence, and Comorbidity: Results from the National

Survey of Adolescents." *Journal of Counseling and Clinical* Psychology 71, no. 4: 692–700.

Kosack, Godula. 2004. "Adopting a Native Child: An Anthropologist's Personal Involvement in the Field." In *Cross-Cultural Approaches to Adoption*, edited by F. Bowie, 21–29. New York, NY: Routledge.

Leifsen, Esben. 2004. "Person, Relation and Value: The Economy of Circulating Ecuadorian Children in International Adoption." In *Cross-Cultural Approaches to Adoption*, edited by F. Bowie, 182–195. New York, NY: Routledge.

———. 2009 "Adoption and the Governing of Child Welfare in 20th Century Quito." *Journal of Latin American and Caribbean Anthropology* 14, no. 1: 68–91.

Leinaweaver, Jessica B. 2008a. "Improving Oneself: Young People Getting Ahead in the Peruvian Andes." *Latin American Perspectives* 35, no. 4: 60–78.

———. 2008b. *The Circulation of Children: Kinship, Adoption, and Morality in Andean Peru*. Durham, NC: Duke University Press.

———. 2009 "Kinship into the Peruvian Adoption Office: Reproducing Families, Producing the State." *Journal of Latin American and Caribbean* Anthropology 14, no. 1: 44–67.

Leinaweaver, Jessica B. and Linda J. Seligmann. 2009. "Introduction: Cultural and Political Economies of Adoption in Latin America." *Journal of Latin American and Caribbean Anthropology* 14, no. 1: 1–19.

López-Cevallos, Daniel and Chunhuei Chi. 2009. "Health Care Utilization in Ecuador: A Multilevel Analysis of Socio-Economic Determinants and Inequality Issues. Health Policy and Planning." http://www.who.int/pmnch/topics/economics/20091116.

———. 2012a. "Inequity in Health Care Utilization in Ecuador: An Analysis of Current Issues and Potential Solutions." *International Journal for Equity in Health* 11 Supplement 1: A6–A7.

———. 2012b. "Migration, remittances, and health care utilization in Ecuador." *Revista Panamericana de Salud* Pública 31, no. 1: 9–16.

Lygnegård, Frida, Dana Donahue, Juan Bornman, Mats Granlund, and Karina Huus. 2013. "A Systematic Review of Generic and Special Needs of Children with Disabilities Living in Poverty Settings in Low- and Middle-Income Countries." *Journal of Policy Practice* 12, no. 4: 296–315.

Marre, Diana and Laura Briggs, eds. 2009 *International Adoption: Global Inequalities and the Circulation of Children*. New York: New York University Press.

McKenzie, Judith K. 1993. "Adoption of Children with Special Needs." *Adoption* 3, no. 1: 62–76.

Melås, Maria Kristine José, Olvind Kvello, and Monica Dalen. 2014. "Internationally Adopted Children after Arrival: Temperament, Behavior Problems, and Age at Adoption as Predictors of Early Motor and Communication Competence." *Adoption Quarterly* 17, no. 1: 28–43.

Mental Disability Rights International. 2004. "Human Rights & Mental Health in Peru." http://www.disabilityrightsintl.org/wordpress/wp-content/uploads/Peru-Report-Eng-Final.pdf Published collaboratively with *Asociación Pro Derechos Humanos*.

Minetti, Alberto, Sandro Galea, and Ezra Susser. 2012. "Community Mental Health Services in Latin America for People with Severe Mental Disorders." *Public Health Reviews* 34, no. 2: 1–23.

Minnis, Helen, Kimberley Everett, Anthony J. Pelosi, Judy Dunn, and Martin Knapp. 2006. "Children in Foster Care: Mental Health, Service Use and Costs." *European Child & Adolescent Psychiatry* 15, no. 2: 63–70.

Newberry, Jan. 2009. "The Circulation of Children: Kinship, Adoption, and Morality in Andean Peru by Jessaca Leinaweaver." *International Journal of Sociology of the Family* 35, no. 2: 209–211.

Oswald, Sylvia H., Katharina Heil, and Lutz Goldbeck. 2010. "History of Maltreatment and Mental Health Problems in Foster Children: A Review of the Literature." *Journal of Pediatric Psychology* 35, no. 5: 462–472.

Pasztor, Eileen Mayers, David Swanson Hollinger, Moira Inkelas, and Neal Halfon. 2006. "Health and Mental Health Services for Children in Foster Care: The Central Role of Foster Parents." *Child Welfare* 85, no. 1: 33–57.

Pérez-Escamillia, Rafael and Hugo Melgar-Quiñonez, eds. 2011 *At Risk: Latino Children's Health*. Houston: Arte Público Press.

Redacción Justicia. 2012. "'Muchos gays quieren adoptar en Colombia y no pueden': Chandler Burr." http://www.eltiempo.com/archivo/documento/CMS-11865445

Rosenthal, James A. 1993. "Outcomes of Adoption of Children with Special Needs." *Adoption* 3, no. 1: 77–88.

Roy, Ranjan. 2011. *Social Support, Health, and Illness: A Complicated Relationship*. Buffalo, NY: University of Toronto Press.

Salazar, Ximena, Clara Sandoval Figureoa, J. Maziel Girón, and Carlos F. Cáceres. 2009. "Gender, Masculinities and HIV/AIDS: Perspectives from Peru." In *Gender and HIV/AIDS: Critical Perspectives from the Developing World*, edited by J. Boesten and Nana K. Poky, 47–66. Burlington, VT: Ashgate Publishing Company.

Sar, Bibhuti K. 2000. "Preparation for Adoptive Parenthood with a Special-Needs Child." *Adoption Quarterly* 3, no. 4: 63–80.

Selman, Peter. 2004. "Adoption: A Cure for Too Many Ills?". In *Cross-Cultural Approaches to Adoption*, edited by F. Bowie, 257–273. New York, NY: Routledge.

Somma, D., B.E. Thomas, F. Karim, J. Kepmp, N. Arias, C. Auer, G.D. Gosoniu, A. Abouihia, and M.G. Weiss. 2008. "Gender and Socio-Cultural Determinants of TB-Related Stigma in Bangladesh, India, Malawi and Colombia." *International Journal of Tuberculosis and Lung Disease* 12, no. 7: 856–866.

Sonne, Paul. 2014. "Russia Tightens Anti-Gay Adoption Ban: Singles from Countries where Gay Marriage Legal Not Allowed to Adopt." http://online.wsj.com/news/articles/SB10001424052702304434104579380613782162016?mg=reno64-wsj&url=http percent3A percent2F percent2Fonline.wsj.com percent2Farticle percent2FSB10001424052702304434104579380613782162016.html.

Stillwaggon, Eileen. 2000 HIV Transmission in Latin America: Comparison with Africa and Policy Implications. *South African Journal of Economics* 68, no. 5: 444–454.

U.S. Department of State. 2014a. "Ecuador." http://adoption.state.gov/country_information/country_specific_info.php?country-select=ecuador.

U.S. Department of State. 2014b. "Colombia." http://adoption.state.gov/country_information/country_specific_info.php?country-select=colombia.

UNAIDS. 2012. "Ecuadorian Government Implements Social Protection Policy for Children Living with HIV." 2014. http://www.unaids.org/en/resources/presscentre/featurestories/2012/october/20121003aecuador/.

Van Dorn, Richard, Jan Volavka, and Norman Johnson. 2012. "Mental Disorder and Violence: Is There a Relationship Beyond Substance Use?" *Social Psychiatry and Psychiatric Epidemiology* 47, no. 3: 487–503.

van IJzendoorn, Marinus H., Femmie Juffer, and Caroline W. Klein Poelhuis. 2005. "Adoption and Cognitive Development: A Meta-Analytic Comparison of Adopted and Nonadopted Children's IQ and School Performance." *Psychological Bulletin* 131, no. 2: 301–316.

van London, W. Monique, Femmie Juffer, and Marinus H. van IJzendoorrn. 2007. "Attachment, Cognitive, and Motor Development in Adopted Children: Short-term Outcomes after International Adoption." *Journal of Pediatric Psychology* 32, no. 10: 1249–1258.

Van Vleet, Krista E. 2002 "The Intimacies of Power: Rethinking Violence and Affinity in the Bolivian Andes." *American Ethnologist* 29, no. 3: 567–601.

———. 2009. "'We Had Already Come to Love Her': Adoption at the Margins of the Bolivian State." *Journal of Latin American and Caribbean Anthropology* 14, no. 1: 20–43.

van Wichelen, Sonja. 2014. "Medicine as Moral Technology: Somatic Economies and the Making Up of Adoptees." *Medical Anthropology: Cross-Cultural Studies in Health and Illness* 33, no. 2: 109–127.

Vandebroek, Ina, Jan-Bart Calewaert, Stijn De jonckheere, Sabino Sanca, Lucio Semo, Patrick Van Damme, Luc Van Puyvelde, and Norbert De Kimpe. 2004. "Use of Medicinal Plants and Pharmaceuticals by Indigenous Communities in the Bolivian Andes and Amazon." *Bulletin of the World Health Organization* 82, no. 4: 243–250.

Waldman, H. Barry, Steven P. Perlman, and Rick Rader. 2010. "Hardships of Raising Children with Special Health Care Needs (A Commentary)." *Social Work in Health Care* 49, no. 7: 618–629.

Wright, Shelley Elizabeth. 2012. *Toward the Mouth of the Abyss: The Indigenous Nature of Cleft Lip and Palate*. Depth Psychology, Pacifica Graduate Institute.

Chapter Eight

"Here to Stay in the Bay!"

The Politics of Vestibularity, Black Trans Women of Jamaica, Gendered Duress, and the Work of Recognition

Antwann Michael Simpkins†

On July 21, 2013 Montego Bay, the capital of Saint James parish in Jamaica, reached a temperature of ninety-three degrees Fahrenheit (NKJS 2013). While ninety-three degrees was a considerably warm day for those residing in the Caribbean nation, the day's summer temperature fell just short of matching the record of ninety-five degrees set in 2002, yet it was higher than the average of eighty-seven degrees (NKJS 2013.). As the sun set on the island a native of Jamaica, Gully Queen, and two of her close friends, Khloe and Keke, decided they would enjoy an evening out in the Irwin community of the Saint James parish as the temperature had cooled to seventy-six degrees (NKJS 2013; McFadden 2013). Seemingly to avoid crowds in an effort to protect themselves Gully Queen, Khloe, and Keke headed out under the cover of Jamaica's late night. The insight of the group to leave at a time that would allow them some measure of protection by avoiding crowds was a lesson well-learned via a long history of cisgender-hetero-masculine violence from citizens of the island nation. As trans women, Gully Queen, Khloe, and Keke were familiar with the many mob attacks against those who occupied Jamaican space and did not identify as heterosexual or present as cisgender.[1] The concerns of the women may have been additionally elevated due to the fact that Javed Jaghai, a gay young man of Jamaica who graduated from Dartmouth College in the United States, filed a complaint on February 7, 2013 with the Supreme Court of Jamaica (*Huffington Post*, February 2, 2013). Jaghai's complaint challenged Jamaica's anti-sodomy law and was soon to be adjudicated (*Huffington Post*, February 2, 2013). The legal complaint became the cause of increasing anti-LGBTQIA rhetoric and threats, physical violence against LGBTQIA community members of Jamaica, as well as Jaghai's family, and himself, being threatened (*The Gleaner*, August 29, 2014). Jaghai's

Supreme Court complaint was grounded in his landlord evicting him due to his sexual orientation (Lavers 2013). Jaghai's predicament may have resonated with Gully Queen, Khloe, and Keke as they resided in an abandoned government house in Albion because their families and communities excommunicated them as well (McFadden).

As this was taking place, Jamaica was experiencing a surging murder rate, as well as increasing acts of violence toward women and girls (Amnesty International 2015). This phenomenon was further compounded by the killing of twenty-one people by police officers in a matter of six days just a few months earlier. These twenty-one deaths at the hands of the State were emblematic of police violence taking place across the island nation. In 2013, police killed on average about five people a week. Between 2000 and 2010 "more than 2,200 fatal shootings by police" had been reported; however, "only two police officers have been convicted for their involvement in killings, according to Amnesty International."[2] Gully Queen, Khloe, and KeKe's decision to use the cover of night to travel may have also been further informed by Gully Queen's previous encounter with the police when they threatened to shoot her. Whatever their reasoning, the women understood they were not safe among civilian men and police officers, and would soon come to learn their cisgender-hetero sisters were not a safe haven, as well.

Arriving shortly after 2 a.m., Gully Queen, Khloe, and Keke entered the local town bar as common bar-goers—participating as accepted community members who danced away the coming worries of a soon-to-be Monday (McFadden). Gully Queen quickly became the center of attention among the several men who were at the bar. As night transitioned into early morning the inside of the riverside bar was filled with laughs, sweat, and dance as the music tinged an otherwise quiet roadside passageway. Gully Queen's dancing rivaled the dancing of other women in attendance. Her skilled and practiced movement paired well with her long legs and high cheekbones. She was a hit—combining splits, dutty wining, nuanced footwork, and other intricate rhythmic choreographies that signified everything from the sociocultural history of the African Diaspora to the syncopated rhythms of Jamaican dancehall music.[3]

As Gully Queen danced she transformed from ostracized Other to community member; for her, dancing meant recognition, belonging, and citizenship. Dance, for Gully Queen, mitigated the psychological impact of her high school experience as a pariah. During the July late night/early morning gathering she was praised for being a skilled and capable woman. Those gathered at the bar were not driven to expel her from the neighborhood as they did years earlier, with the help of her parents, when she was fourteen years old. For the time being, she was not a refugee among her own—rather, her community accepted her. Nearly three hundred members of her community affirmed her as she danced (McFadden). Dance for Gully Queen was more than merriment, it was the choreography of citizenship—granting her proper recognition, inclusion, and her being counted as one among the many.

As she danced, a resident of the Irwin community paid particular attention to Gully Queen's features. Soon the woman, by way of her subjective cognition, recognized Gully Queen as a young male who at one point had attended the same church as she did (Brown 2013). The church-going woman began to inform patrons of the bar, particularly the men, that the skilled woman who was the center of attention was a male. Soon Gully Queen was surrounded by men who were friends of the church-going woman. As the men closed in on Gully Queen, the interior space of the bar illuminated as the flame from a lighter expelled the darkness of the coming morning, delineating citizen from Other. The men inspected Gully Queen's body, determining that her feet were "too large to belong to a woman" (Associated Press 2013). While Gully Queen's feet were examined, another patron grabbed a lantern, shining its light on Gully Queen from crown to foot (Associated Press 2013). The crowd of cisgender men and women quickly grew enraged. With the cover of darkness interrupted by butane fire, Gully Queen was immediately refused her womanhood and simultaneously denied manhood—she became an ungendered liminal being whereby cisgender men and women in attendance at the bar understood themselves and their rights in relation to her being; she became vestibular.[4]

As the crowd's anger and contempt grew, Khloe whispered in Gully Queen's ear "walk with me, walk with me" (Associated Press 2013). Gully Queen, refusing Khloe's request, informed those at the bar that she was a woman. As she declared her gender identity and her truth, Gully Queen felt a snap-like sensation from behind. A person in the crowd attempted to grab her from behind, causing her bra to break—Gully Queen, knowing that her death may be imminent, panicked and ran (Associated Press 2013); the crowd quickly followed her. At sixteen years old, Gully Queen was beaten, stabbed, shot, and run over by a car (McFadden). Khloe was also beaten, and was sexually assaulted; however she found shelter in a church after being raped (Associated Press). Keke, although scraped, escaped (Associated Press 2013).

When Gully Queen's father received news of what had transpired, he refused to identify her body (McFadden). Instead, Gully Queen's queer family, Khloe and Keke, identified the body of the once-spirited and lively teen who lived in bushes, on the beach, and in abandoned government houses (Associated Press). Although nearly 300 people were at the bar that fateful July morning in Montego Bay, no one has provided police with the names of those who murdered Gully Queen.

"THEY'LL JUST KILL US FASTER"

When cisgender-hetero acts of violence such as that which happened to Gully Queen take place, it wills me to contemplate how numerous citizens of Jamaica come to view specific human lives as worthy of communal excommunication, violence, and death. The narrative of Gully Queen also compels a consideration of the ways in which law works to construct citizens, afford rights, and inform protest movements. This chapter attempts to address this question while simultaneously illuminating a few of the many ways Jamaican law prohibits specific representations of gender and sexuality, thereby causing the societal rejection of trans persons as possible citizens as well as the production and reproduction of gendered duress. Of importance to this work are the social, political, and legal terrains of Jamaica. Specifically, I give attention to how law in Jamaica positions, constructs, and articulates hetero(sexuality) as normative and essential to nation building (and thus a requisite for citizenship), while simultaneously positioning queer identities, specifically impoverished Black trans women, as both central and antithetical to the Jamaican State.[5]

Gendered duress "is a choreography of law which imposes forced conditions of confinement, the persistent threat of a harm, and/or the constraining of rights and the hidden injury that Black women experience" (Simpkins 2016). More specifically, gendered duress is defined as choreography because "it is a carefully crafted dance of disavowal and universalism in which violations are not acknowledged by law as illegal or injurious until it is mapped onto white bodies; it is lawful[ly] permitted bia[s] resulting in the penalization of both a racialized and gendered status as opposed to conduct" (Simpkins 2016). However, in Jamaica gendered duress manifests differently—it becomes recognized when it occurs among wealthy queer individuals, as gully queens remain "impoverished, without the support of their families and larger society, and without prospects of finding a job" (Frank 2016). Jamaica's gully queens are "constantly subjected to hateful acts of violence, [that is] solely enacted on the basis of prejudice and animosity" and their socioeconomic status, forcing them to live in the "dark corners of public spaces, where resources are scarce and danger is a constant threat" thus perpetually exposing them to gendered duress (Frank 2016).

When the laws of Jamaica are critically examined what becomes immediately apparent is systematically poor trans women in Jamaica, like the enslaved Black women Hortense Spillers centers in her work, are "the principal point of passage between the human and non-human world" (2003, 155). Concerning enslaved Black women Spillers advances they are "the focus of a cunning difference—visually, psychologically, ontologically—as the route by which dominant modes decided the distinction between humanity and 'other.' At this radical level of discontinuity in the 'great chain of being,' black is vestibular to culture. In other words, the black person mirrored for society around her what a human being was not" (Spillers 2003).

When the lives of Black trans women in Jamaica are taken seriously in scholarship as well as in the work of justice not only does Spillers's assertion remain true, but we are also able to map the intimate and isolated space of Spiller's vestibular beyond what we currently know it to be. As a result, vestibularity, along with being "the route by which dominant modes decide the distinction between humanity and 'other'" (Spillers 2003), also comes to be a legally constructed corporeal locale of violence, dispossession, coerced ungendering, sub-humanness, and communal exclusion, as well as the place of production for the requisites of citizenship and proper recognition in society. The vestibular as corporeal, in this sense, is both centered in society and marginal; the trans body, via law, is conscribed to act as the defining line of who is a citizen and who is not. Further, the trans subject as vestibular comes to indicate who belongs at the margins of society and why, while concomitantly mapping the terrain of the public sphere, constructing the sociopolitical composition of the nation and its attending societal benefits, and defining the outermost limits of society, as well as dictating the terms of interpersonal engagement among society. In so many words to be vestibular is to be simultaneously ontological, epistemological, and political, while being the site of production for the social and political identities which are recognized as legitimate in society. Indeed Danielle Allen in *Talking to Strangers* offers "political order is secured not only by institutions, but also by 'deep rules' that prescribe specific interactions among citizens in public spaces; citizens enact what they are to each other not only in assemblies, where they make decisions about their mutually intertwined fates, but also when, as strangers, they speak to one another, or don't, or otherwise respond to each other's presence" (2004, 10). Differently stated, the citizen-self is defined in relation to the socially-aberrant Other who, in this instance, are poor Black trans women.

As law works to produce liminal subjects, and thus their otherness resulting in the production of vestibular beings, those persons encounter unyielding State violence. However, vestibularity should not be primarily understood as a location of violent dispossession. As the State acts upon vestibular beings, the vestibular as corporeal also becomes the site of radical protest and refusal—thus exposing the tension between being constructed as Other versus not conceiving of oneself as Other. While gully queens do live in open sewer passages, abandoned government homes, and other public spaces, those spaces are nonetheless being occupied by those whom the State rejects. In other words, the Rejected occupying the propertied spaces of government constitutes an act of organized protest. Said another way, the gully queens of Jamaica allow for an understanding that the vestibular is also a location comprised of a dissident culture where dance, coded language, and collective community (among many other things) merge in order to contest societal rejection by means of what anthropologist James C. Scott terms infrapolitics—"the circumspect struggle waged daily by subordinate groups . . . beyond the visible end of the spectrum. That it should be invisible . . . is in large part by design—a tactical choice born of a prudent awareness of the balance of power" (1990, 183). Indeed historian Robin Kelley affirms the use of infrapolitics among oppressed groups describing it as "the daily confrontations, evasive actions, and stifled thoughts that often inform organized political movements" (1994, 8).

Beyond gender identity, the narrative of Gully Queen also compels us to consider how class impacts the lived experiences of Black trans women in Jamaica. While Gully Queen was known by her name she belonged to a community known as the gully queens—queer youth of color who live in the sewer passages, bushes, beaches, and abandoned government homes of Jamaica. This group of youth are noticeably different from Jamaica's "rich queens"—queer persons who are exceptionally wealthy, and thus, are often protected from public anti-queer violence. As a result, gully queens come to experience gendered duress because their persisting injury is both produced and reproduced by the convergence of law and capitalism, yet unacknowledged by it.

The gully queens of Jamaica understand both their sociopolitical and economic positioning and predicament clearly, as well as its implications. When a queer individual was recently asked in an interview if they thought Jamaica would ever evolve regarding its cultural understanding and treatment of Jamaican queer persons they responded, "It's never going to happen. They'll just kill us faster" (Frank). Directing our attention to the lived experiences of gully queens in Jamaica is important because we should know their stories and struggles with the State, and because gully queens complicate our understanding of the trans experience in Jamaica—as their lives "reject the idea of static, monolithic, bounded categories" concerning trans persons among the citizenry (Cohen 1997, 441). Indeed some trans women, "rich-queens," and trans men are able to negotiate public space without fear due to their ability to pass.[6] Furthermore, they are also protected from the persistent and intrusive surveillance of the public by way of the location of their homes. Both of these characteristics reflect and reinforce the heteronormative expectations of society; however, more importantly, they are only experienced due to the economic positioning of the individual. In other words, what the lives of "rich queens" in Jamaica evidence is, as Cathy Cohen argues, "the ways in which varying relations to power exist not only among heterosexuals, but also among those who label themselves queer" (1997, 449). Therefore, class and/or material privilege simultaneously informs the capacity to navigate public space safely as a rich queen and the protest efforts of Jamaica's gully queens.

Gully Queen is not alone in her torment and murder at the hands of anonymous cisgender men and women disguised in the carefully constructed and guarded shroud of toxic hetero-masculine patriarchy. Rather, Gully Queen's lived experience reflects the many queer lives of Jamaica that have been assaulted and killed in unspeakable and unfathomable ways. However, those who lived to tell their story refuse to remain perpetual victims to toxic hetero-masculinity or to let experiences such as that of Gully Queen be wholly claimed by anti-trans violence and rhetoric. For queer persons in Jamaica, the personal is both political and a call to protest. Toward this end, this work also explores sites of queer protests in Jamaica in an effort to illuminate hetero-masculinity's inability to kill us all, as it explores the nation's harmful and discriminative laws.

"Throwing bottles, stones, and other missiles"

> 76. Whosoever shall be convicted of the abominable crime of buggery, committed either with mankind or with any animal, shall be liable to be imprisoned and kept to hard labor for a term not exceeding ten years. (Offences Against the Person Act 1876)
>
> 77. Whosoever shall attempt to commit the said abominable crime, or shall be guilty of any assault with intent to commit the same, or of any indecent assault upon any male person, shall be guilty of a misdemeanor, and being convicted thereof, shall be liable to be imprisoned for a term not exceeding seven years. (Offences Against the Person Act 1876)
>
> 79. Any male person who, in public or private, commits, or is a party to the commission by any male person of, any act of gross indecency with another male person, shall be guilty of a misdemeanor, and being convicted thereof shall be liable at the discretion of the court to be imprisoned for a term not exceeding two years, with or without hard labor. (Offences Against the Person Act 1876)

As Jamaica gained its independence, the expectations of gender performance and sexual expression remained as it had under British rule. The continued use of the anti-buggery laws within the Offences Against the Person Act, often leads many to conclude that Jamaica's anti-queer stance is a product of colonialism. However, an examination of early Caribbean societies proves otherwise. Historian, Kathleen Phillips Lewis provides "gender role differentiation and oppression of women were deeply entrenched in indigenous island societies and was not simply a European phenomenon imposed from the outside" (1993, 9). Phillips Lewis further advances "gender oppression in Caribbean indigenous societies took form sometimes akin to its outer-world counterparts, but in other respects was so totally indigenous that it baffled European observers" (1993; see note).[7] In other words, before, as well as during and after, the colonialization of Jamaica anti-queer cisgender-male-hetero politic was essential to both the formation of Jamaican society and meaning making on the island.

As laws were established and retained in the nation, particularly those outlining sexual behaviors deemed normative in Jamaica, the bodies and intimate lives of queer persons became illegal, surveilled, and marginalized. Jamaica's anti-buggery laws, established in 1864, came to have the effect of codifying heterosexuality and interpreting the norms of heterosexuality through the lives of non-hetero persons—although their lives remained silenced as the lens by which gender normativity was established. The anti-buggery laws' specific attention to queer persons positioned non-cisgender and non-hetero persons as sociopolitical vestibulars, wherein their lives came to define the limits of gender and sexual normativity in Jamaica. Moreover, these laws communicated to those deemed normative citizens in Jamaica that the lives of queer persons are antithetical to Jamaican society as well as a threat to the island as a nation. The retention of these laws in postcolonial Jamaica indicate, as M. Jaqui Alexander argues concerning Trinidad and Tobago and the Bahamas, that Jamaica when it "move[d] to reconfigure the nation" as it gained its independence from Britain simultaneously worked to "resuscitate the nation as hetero*sexual*" (Alexander 1994, 6).

Therefore, Jamaicans who are queer are understood to be unworthy of citizenship to the point of disposability, injury, and violent exclusion. In 2011, two years before Gully Queen's brutal murder, twenty well-equipped police officers executed a raid on a club in Montego Bay which the queer community of Jamaica built for themselves. Approaching the nightclub, which was filled with unsuspecting queer patrons, police officers "jumped from their vehicles, aggressively accosting patrons, kicking in doors, beating and pistol whipping indiscriminately, and chasing everyone from the venue" (White 2013). Those that were at the Montego Bay club reported that police officers were verbally insulting the patrons as they were physically attacked and also called for party-goers at other clubs in the surrounding area to "join in the melee by throwing bottles, stones, and other missiles" (White 2013). The police raid on the club demonstrates the close relationship between the Jamaican State and hetero-sexuality and normativity, yet also evidences that violence against queer persons is both a social phenomenon and is perceived to be a responsibility of citizenship which cisgender-hetero identifying persons are expected to perform. This point becomes salient when reflecting on the 2002 political campaign year in Jamaica.

In 2002, the leading political parties of Jamaica grounded their campaigns in queer-antagonistic music and refused to abolish or challenge the nation's anti-buggery laws. The Jamaican Labour Party selected T.O.K's "Chi Chi Man" as its theme song, while the People's National Party theme of "Log On to Progress" was inspired by Elephant Man's hit single "Log On." Both "Chi Chi Man" and "Log On" are popular Jamaican reggae tracks composed of lyrics which advocate the harm of queer persons (White 2013). These acts of violent exclusion and political marginalization make it clear that "not just (any) *body* can be a citizen any more . . . *some* bodies have been marked by the [S]tate as non-procreative, in pursuit of sex only for pleasure, a sex that is non-productive of babies and of no economic gain" and, as a result, come to constitute "a profound threat to the very survival of the nation" (Alexander).

Although the sociopolitical environment of Jamaica is harmful and injurious for all queer persons residing on the island, it is particularly dangerous and violent for impoverished Black trans women. In 2016 a trans woman and her friends stopped at a gas station after attending an event at National Stadium in Kingston. After leaving the gas station "a vehicle carrying a group of men stopped in front of them, blocking them from driving off. Almost immediately, another vehicle blocked them from behind. The men in the front car alighted from their vehicle and pulled the transgender woman from her car. They beat her severely, then took her to an inner city community where she was beaten again. The attackers then threw her body in the Sandy Park Gully in St. Andrew and left her for dead" (Human Rights Committee 2016, 4). The report does not indicate what happened to the friends who were accompanying her that evening; however, what is known is the men fixed their attention on the trans woman within the group and accosted her specifically. Fortunately, after her violent encounter, the trans woman (who remains nameless in the report) was spotted by a passerby who called for help. She was taken to the hospital suffering from a "fractured right arm and wounds on her face, arm, hips, and back" (Human Rights Committee 2016).

External physical injury represents only one of the many acts of violence impoverished Black trans women experience in Jamaica. Like their lesbian sisters, trans women also experience "corrective rape" as Khloe had, the evening of Gully Queen's murder. However, in Jamaica trans women cannot be raped as the nation's law limits the recognition of such a violent act to the biological sex category of female and hetero-coerciveness. In this way trans women come to experience gendered duress as they are refused redress when they are raped and, furthermore, are prevented from speaking out as Jamaica's anti-buggery laws, which demand gender-sex alignment, subject trans women to both prison and further multiplied injuries as a result of their incarceration. These instances of murder, bodily injury, and rape evidence impoverished Black trans women are consistently surveilled, denied the privileges of citizenship, and consigned to a specific liminal space wherein their lives become the sacrifice for the exercise of democracy within the nation. Thus, Black trans women within the cisgender-hetero gaze in Jamaica are vital to the nation, as trans women are fashioned into vestibular subjects, via the State, and positioned as sociopolitical interlocutors while at the same time constituting the sacrifice required for democratic productivity and citizenship within Jamaica. Political theorist Danielle Allen argues "as citizens struggle over political questions . . . the site of sacrifice is between the social world . . . and the political world of institutions"; moreover, Allen posits ". . . people who benefit less than others from particular political decisions, but nonetheless accede to those decisions, preserve the stability of political institutions. Their sacrifice makes collective democratic action possible . . . the hard truth of democracy is that some citizens are always giving things up for others" (2004, 28–29). The site of sacrifice between the social world and political institutions which Allen refers to is the location of the trans-vestibular subject where unspeakable acts of violence are unacknowledged by law and are permitted to take place. This allows for an understanding that while trans women are marginal in Jamaican society, they are also central to it, in that within the gaze of cisgender-hetero and/or favorably classed Jamaican citizens impoverished Black trans women, as well as other queer identified persons, come to define for the cisgender-hetero and class-privileged citizens of the island nation who they understand themselves to be and the rights to which they are entitled to.

The gaze of the privileged class within Jamaica, in turn, then comes to animate the political and social power dynamics among the populace of the island. These power dynamics are critical as they translate to resource politics—meaning who has the right to participate in the claiming of resources and to what extent. These power dynamics also act to solidify who is recognized as a citizen of Jamaica as well as who may navigate the public spaces of Jamaica as a trans person. Most importantly, the gendered and class power dynamics of Jamaica superimpose onto the lives of impoverished trans women and queer persons the weight of democratic sacrifice. An area in which the weight of democratic sacrifice as well as the gendered and class dynamics of Jamaica come into sharp relief is health care.

THE PERSONAL IS POLITICAL

Poor trans women in Jamaica are severely limited in their access to proper health care. As vestibular subjects poor trans women are seen neither as legitimate citizens, nor as women in need of specific forms of care like their cisgender-hetero sisters or their wealthy trans sisters and brothers. Instead, impoverished trans women of Jamaica are persistently marginalized and exposed to gendered duress in its many forms as they remain silently centered within Jamaican political consciousness.[8] While most health-care reports concerning trans women focus on the urgent need for proper HIV/AIDS care, what is given less attention is the enduring psychological trauma poor trans women experience, as well as the types of reproductive care trans women need. The failure of most health-care professionals and public officials in Jamaica to recognize these needs is not surprising; interestingly, evidence suggests it is intentional. Indeed Melissa Harris-Perry in her text *Sister Citizen* advances, "an individual who is seen primarily as a part of a despised group loses the opportunity to experience the public recognition for which the human self strives. Further, if the group itself is misunderstood, then to the extent that one is seen as part of this group, that 'seeing' is inaccurate. Inaccurate recognition is painful not only to the psyche but also to the political self, the citizen self" (2011, 38).

For some it is difficult to map how reproductive rights are implicated in the lives of trans women. At the core of reproductive rights is the ability of women to determine what happens to their bodies, as well as how and when it happens. More often than not the understanding of the ability to choose is grounded primarily in the decision (not) to birth a child. However, this approach to reproductive rights is limiting in that it recognizes women as citizens and their access to rights (or lack thereof) via the productivity of their wombs. However, when the Reproductive Health Survey for Jamaica is reviewed, it yields a different understanding of what we know reproductive rights and care to be.

The questionnaire for "females" included in the 2008 Jamaican Reproductive Health Survey asks citizens who are women several questions: which parish they belong to; the number of persons in their household; do they attend religious services; what they did during the past week; if they work; do they read newspapers; what type of technology they have in their home; what is the main source of water for their home; the type of toilet they use in their home; and if they are legally married; among several other questions (National Family Planning Board 2010; see note).[9] What these questions suggest is that Jamaican authorities are aware reproductive rights and care encompass more than the womb. Rather, reproductive rights and care are also about the extent to which someone is connected to their community; their access to jobs and information; and their access to adequate resources to properly maintain their hygiene. This allows for the understanding that in Jamaica, reproductive rights and care are about the holistic well-being of women, not just the moments in which women choose to (or not to) have children. In other words, what Jamaica understands is that women contribute to their communities in various ways beyond childbirth; and that whichever way women choose to contribute to their communities that contribution is (and should be) valued, surveyed, protected, and quantified so as to guarantee both the access to the means to produce the contribution as well as the continuation of the contribution with the support of the Jamaican State apparatus and society.

Insightfully, the survey also asks: "are you and your husband currently living together as husband and wife?"; "are you currently living with a common-law partner? That is, are you living as husband and wife with a partner to whom you are not legally married?"; "do you currently have a visiting partner? That is, do you have a steady partner with whom you have sexual relations?"; "do you currently have a boyfriend?"; "have you ever had sexual intercourse with your current boyfriend?"; "have you ever been in a partnership; that is, a marriage, a common-law union or visiting union?"; and "how many times have you been in a partnership; that is, a marriage, a common-law union, or a visiting union?" (National Family Planning Board 2010). Exploring these questions along with those previously stated are important in that they reveal government officials are also cognizant that there are several different ways in which one may choose to facilitate family beyond traditional marriage, and that a familial formation may or may not include intercourse ("have you ever had sexual intercourse with your boyfriend?").

What these questions, as well as many others, on the questionnaire reveal is the womb is only one aspect of reproductive rights and care. These questions suggest the availability of jobs are just as important as women's wombs; that the many ways in which family may be facilitated is, in fact, important to the nation; that one's connection to one's community is equally important as one's risk of contracting HIV/AIDS; and that an individual's access to owning a home is just as important as regular visits to the doctor. Yet in all of these areas impoverished Black trans women in Jamaica face steep barriers because the nation grounds its policies in gender-sex alignment—which works to simultaneously privilege cisgender women and punish trans women, particularly those who are poor, because of their status.

As impoverished Black trans women live in the gullies of various parishes, they are simultaneously prevented from accessing gainful employment due to societal stigma. When impoverished Black trans women form families, similar to Gully Queen, Keke, and Khloe, their differing familial formations are not acknowledged by the State. When trans women choose to (or choose not to) engage in intimate bonds with their partners, their access to condoms and contraception is not of communal importance and concern similar to that of their cisgender-hetero sisters. The recognition of the right to both access and attain these resources and several others is what it means for impoverished Black trans women in Jamaica to have access to reproductive rights and care.

Combined, these essential resources dovetail to promote the general health of an individual or prevent it by way of social stigmatization and exclusion. In this way the Jamaican State has sentenced queer persons, indeed impoverished Black trans women, to a slow and painful death by way of willful exclusion, intentional political misrecognition, and the refusal of life-preserving resources.[10] While Jamaica's approach to gendered needs allows for an expansive understanding of reproductive rights, the nation's articulation of reproductive rights is constructed in such a way that these rights come to police the boundaries of "woman" through gender-sex-performance alignment—thereby resulting in who is acknowledged as "woman" being carefully constructed and protected. Hence, the State production of the category of "woman," as well as other fixed-gender designations in the island nation, as Sarah Haley argues in her text concerning Black women in U.S. carceral institutions, requires violence (2016, 8). However, despite various State-imposed and socially perpetuated obstacles, gully queens remain present and refuse to "go away with [their] issues of sexuality"; instead, they are coming home (Hemphill 1992).

On October 25, 2015, Keke stood draped in a rainbow flag which she had fashioned into a dress. This time she was not running in fear for her life. Instead, with her head crowned with colorful flowers, she stood confident, holding a microphone in her right hand, as clouds passed over a humid seventy-nine-degree Fall night in the St. James Parish of Montego Bay (TimeandDate.com 2015). Keke was taking part in constructing and fortifying her family and community. She was claiming the reproductive rights and care which had been denied her by the State. Her presence signaled to the community gathered at the Talent & Fashion show during Montego Bay's first pride event, that despite the State-sponsored death of Gully Queen she witnessed in July of 2013, gully queens, as a community, two years later were still present and refused to be silenced or moved; instead they decided to occupy various sites owned by the State until they received full recognition as citizens in Jamaica—even if it meant residing in the gullies of the island nation.

Montego Bay's first pride was organized under the motto of "Here to Stay in the Bay!"[11] The events of the pride were as much an act of community building as it was organized protests. Four years earlier in 2011, before taking office as Prime Minister, Portia Simpson-Miller "opposed discrimination against LGBT people and indicated a willingness to review the country's criminali[z]ation" of queer persons (Writer 2015). Her efforts materialized as the Charter of Fundamental Rights and Freedoms. However, the anticipated charter, similar to the Offences Against the Person Act, grounded its protections in biological deterministic prose: "the right to freedom from discrimination on the ground of—(i) being male or female. . . ." Intentionally left out of the 2011 parliamentary legislation were explicit protections for queer persons living in Jamaica (Charter of Fundamental Rights and Freedoms 2011). After having their hopes dashed yet again, queer organizations began to mobilize, erecting places of refuge and providing the resources and protections which the State of Jamaica disallowed.

J-FLAG, Jamaica's most prominent voice in queer advocacy, began establishing shelters for queer Jamaican youth. The National Anti-Discrimination Alliance began providing both safe houses and private shelters for queer Jamaican citizens. The establishment of these centers are both life-preserving work and simultaneously direct protest against the State: as of 2015, Jamaica has experienced a 26 percent rise in its homeless population; of this figure 40 percent are queer youth (Rezvany 2016). These shelters also attend to the health needs of queer individuals as there is a "high occurrence of HIV and other medical problems within the long-term LGBTQ homeless community, as well as a high rate of unemployment and training" (Rezvany 2016). In addition to these disparities, LGBTQIA persons in Jamaica live with persisting psychological trauma. A community organizer who does community work in shelters and safe homes disclosed "they've been traumatized. Re-traumatized. And traumatized ten times on top of that" (Rezvany 2016).

J-FLAG and the National Anti-Discrimination Alliance are not alone in their efforts. TransWave, established in August of 2015, addresses the specific needs of trans persons in Jamaica. The organization focuses on "HIV Transmission, health-care access, gender-based violence (GBV) and other social issues that put the community at risk" (TransWave 2015). The organization also gives voice to trans persons and their experiences by chronicling Jamaican trans history, as well as interviewing willing members of the trans community so that "readers may be enlightened about their personal journeys" and that the trans community may develop and maintain a positive-image (TransWave 2015). TransWave refuses to allow the voices of trans persons to be stifled, muted, or controlled. The organization has a strict policy regarding engaging TransWave and the community it represents: "we welcome respectful discussion and reserve the right to moderate or block commenters as we deem fit" (2015).

The work of pride organizers and queer organizations in Jamaica demonstrates the personal is both political and a means of organizing across difference. Whereas the State refuses to acknowledge queer persons, indeed trans women, as citizens or afford them rights, queer persons, in turn, have erected indigenous institutions of their own thereby establishing both community and rights among themselves. What the lives of trans women in Jamaica demonstrate is despite the State's best effort to silence and marginalize their community, they refuse to go away quietly into the night while suffering unspeakable harms unacknowledged by law.

In the official State records we will never know Gully Queen's name. In all State documents and articles concerning Gully Queen, she is ungendered and remade again in masculinity as Dwayne Jones in the State's final act of disavowal. Yet, even here, the personal too is political. A Black woman, who is a Jamaican human rights activist, founded Dwayne's House—a queer friendly shelter—in protest to the State's attempt to co-opt the life and value of Gully Queen to her community.[12] In the final analysis, the work of organizers and impoverished Black trans women of Jamaica reveals the vestibular to be a politically imposed corporeal locale where gendered duress is perpetually experienced. However, their lives also demonstrate the vestibular to be a place of social and political protest; it is not wholly consuming. Rather, it is a site of contestation for those who refuse to die for the sake of a violent hetero-exclusionary democracy.

NOTES

† I would like to thank Kathleen Phillips Lewis (Spelman College), Sarah Haley (UCLA), and Sora Han (UC Irvine) for their assistance, critiques, and guidance with this project. Most importantly, I am indebted to the Black transwomen who have challenged my views and encouraged me at different points in my life and intellectual journey: The Lady Chablis, Vanity Reid Deterville, Madison Hinton, Taylor Zoe Malphurs, and Amiyah Scott. Thank you Gully Queen for daring to live.

1. By cisgender I mean the alignment of how one self-identifies and presents socially with their biological sex. For more on this please see: Julia Serano, "Dismantling Cissexual Privilege," in *Whipping Girl: A Transsexual Woman on Sexism and the Scapegoating of Femininity* (Emeryville: Seal Press, 2007); and Sunnivie Brydum, "The True Meaning of the Word 'Cisgender,'" *Advocate*, July 31, 2005. https://www.advocate.com/transgender/2015/07/31/true-meaning-word-cisgender.

2. See "Jamaica Outraged by Police Killings," *Wales Online*, March 27, 2013. https://www.walesonline.co.uk/news/uk-news/jamaica-outraged-by-police-killings-2044516; and Paul Peachy, "Too Many Deaths in Paradise: Jamaica is awash with Police Shootings and has brought in a British Commissioner to Investigate," *The Independent*, January 28, 2014. https://www.independent.co.uk/news/world/americas/too-many-deaths-in-paradise-jamaica-is-awash-with-police-shootings-and-has-brought-in-a-british-9089068.html; the gender and sexuality of each citizen impacted by police killings during this frame is not known. I point to this phenomenon to illuminate the larger social context in which Black trans women must navigate daily as they develop and execute methods of survival.

3. The Best The Epic Trensetta Part 3, "Gully Queen the legend part 1," filmed March 2013, YouTube Video, 2:51. Posted March 2013. https://www.youtube.com/watch?v=_kzTz04yjAs ; dutty wine is a highly rhythmic dance form originating in Jamaica.

4. Sarah Haley advances "subjects are produced in relation to each other. Just as 'the slave is the object or the ground that makes possible the existence of the bourgeois subject and, by negation or contradistinction, defines liberty, citizenship, and the enclosure of the social body,' black females as others made white women, and by extension or negation, white normative femininity, possible. For these essential reasons, scenes of gendered racial terror in this chapter must be considered in the context of black women's lack of protection, for these 'materialized scene[s] of unprotected female flesh—of female flesh "ungendered"' reveal black women's position as a radical other to the normative female subject position 'woman.'" See Sarah Haley, *No Mercy Here: Gender, Punishment, and the Making of Jim Crow Modernity* (Chapel Hill: The University of North Carolina, 2016).

5. Cathy Cohen's definition of heteronormative is instructive here. She states, "by heteronormative I mean both those localized practices and those centralized institutions which legitimize and privilege heterosexuality and heterosexual relationships as fundamental and 'natural' within society." See Cathy Cohen, "Punks, Bulldaggers, and Welfare Queens: The Radical Potential of Queer Politics?," *GLQ*, vol. 3 (1997): 437–465.

6. By the use of "pass" here I mean those who present as biologically (fe)male in social spaces who are trans. More often than not the ability to "pass" is connected with one's economic positioning as they are able to afford the various processes and material goods required to both present and perform the heteronormative standards of gender. The ability to pass as one's gender identity is similar to how some African Americans passed as white during the Jim Crow era in the United States of America.

7. *See endnote 6*. This is not to suggest European colonization did not have an impact in the lives of women in the Caribbean or everyday Caribbean culture; for more, please see: Kathleen Phillips Lewis "European Stereotypes and the Position of Women in the Caribbean: An Historical Overview," in *Crossroads of Empire: The European-Caribbean Connection, 1492–1992* (Cave Hill: University of West Indies Press, 2000): 64–77.

8. A study conducted by J-FLAG, a Jamaican LGBT advocacy organization, found that from May to August of 2015, 72 percent of the articles published in Jamaica concerning LBT women were about trans women; the majority of the articles were negative and exclusionary in tone. See Paige Andrew, "Media Content Analysis Report on Jamaican LBT Women," J-FLAG, September 2015. http://jflag.org/wp-content/uploads/2014/08/WE-Change-Media-Content-Analysis_September-2015.pdf.

9. "Female" is used here because it is the term referenced in the title of the questionnaire in the survey. The decision of the State to use "female" illustrates the State's intention to distinguish who are to be deemed women; and further, what protections they are entitled to.

10. Black trans women are centered in this work. This is not to suggest there are not trans women of differing ethnicities and/or races who reside in Jamaica. However, the particular ways in which race, gender, sexuality, and class converge in Jamaica

oftentimes cause non-Black, favorably classed trans women to be protected by way of their socioeconomic positioning. Because of this I give specific attention to the lived experiences of marginalized Black trans women who are both misrecognized in the nation and refused the protections their favorably socially positioned non-Black trans sisters enjoy.

11. I have intentionally decided not to mention the names of specific organizers, as their lives are very much under persistent threat and exposed to harm—many queer organizers in Jamaica have been killed for their protest work. Their efforts should be applauded and recognized, while at the same time allowing for anonymity.

12. *See endnote 11.*

WORKS CITED

"About." *TransWave*. https://transwavejamaica.wordpress.com/about/.

Alexander, M. Jaqui. "Not Just (Any) Body Can Be a Citizen: The Politics of Law, Sexuality and Postcoloniality in Trinidad and Tobago and the Bahamas." *Feminist Review*, no. 48 (1994): 5–23.

Allen, Danielle S. *Talking to Strangers: Anxieties of Citizenship since Brown v. Board of Education*. Chicago: University of Chicago Press: 2004.

Associated Press. "Jamaican transgender teen's murder by mob prompts for change, tolerance: 'It was horrible. It was so, so painful.'" *NY Daily News* (New York, NY), August 11, 2013. Accessed April 15, 2014. http://www.nydailynews.com/news/world/transgender-teen-murder-sparks-outcry-jamaica-article-1.1423856.

Brown, Dwayne. "16 Year Old Transgender Murdered in Jamaica: Hated to Death." *Minority Insight*, July 17, 2013. Accessed April 15, 2014. http://www.minority-insight.org/2013/07/17-year-old-transgender-murdered-in.html.

Cohen, Cathy. "Punk, Bulldaggers, and Welfare Queens: The Radical Potential of Queer Politics." *GLQ*, vol. 3 (1997): 437–465.

Frank, Pricilla. "These Are The Fearless LGBTQ Youth Who Live In Jamaica's Sewers," *HuffingtonPost.com*, August 30, 2016. https://www.huffingtonpost.com/entry/christo-geoghegan-gully-queen-photos_us_57c09c34e4b085c1ff29586f.

Haley, Sarah. *No Mercy Here: Gender, Punishment, and the Making of Jim Crow Modernity*. Chapel Hill: University of North Carolina, 2016.

Harris-Perry, Melissa V. *Sister Citizen: Shame, Stereotypes, and Black Women in America*. New Haven: Yale University Press, 2011.

Hemphill, Essex. "If Freud Had Been a Neurotic Colored Woman: Reading Dr. Frances Cress Welsing." In *Ceremonies: Prose and Poetry* by Essex Hemphill. New York: Plume, 1992.

"Human Rights Violations Against Lesbian, Gay, Bisexual, and Transgender (LGBT) People in Jamaica: A Shadow Report." Report Submitted 118th Session of the Human Rights Committee, Geneva, 2016. http://tbinternet.ohchr.org/Treaties/CCPR/Shared percent20Documents/JAM/INT_CCPR_CS JAM_25269_E.pdf.

Igual, Roberto. "Jamaican LGBTIs celebrate 1st Montego Bay Pride." Mamba Online (Johannesburg: South Africa), October 30, 2015. http://www.mambaonline.com/2015/10/30/jamaican-lgbtis-celebrate-1st-montego-bay-pride/.

Jamaica: Justice System Must Be Strengthened for the Effective Protection of Human Rights. London: Amnesty International, May 2015. https://www.amnesty.org/download/Documents/AMR3800042014ENGLISH.pdf.

"Jamaican Gay Man Drops Court Challenge Against Anti-Buggery Law." *Jamaica-gleaner.com*, August 29, 2014. http://jamaica-gleaner.com/power/55113.

"Javed Jaghai, Gay Jamaican Man, Set to Challenge Country's Anti-Sodomy Law." *Huffingtonpost.com*, February 2, 2016. https://www.huffingtonpost.com/2013/02/13/javed-jaghai-gay-jamaica-anti-sodomy-laws-_n_2679242.html.

Kelley, Robin D.G. *Race Rebels: Culture, Politics, and the Black Working Class*. New York: The Free Press, 1994.

Lavers, Michael K. "Gay Jamaican, man challenges country's anti-sodomy law." *Washington Blade* (Washington, D.C.), February 12, 2013. http://www.washingtonblade.com/2013/02/12/gay-jamaican-man-challenges-countrys-anti-sodomy-law/.

Lewis, Kathleen Phillips. "Women in Indigenous Caribbean Island Societies." Lecture, University of the West Indies. St. Augustine, Trinidad, November 1993.

McFadden, David. "In Jamaica, transgender teen murdered by mob." *USA Today* (McLean, Virginia) August 11, 2013. https://www.usatoday.com/story/news/world/2013/08/11/jamaica-transgender-teen-murdered-by-mob/2639995/.

"Past Weather in Montego Bay, Jamaica—October 2015" *Time and Date* (Stavaner, Norway). Accessed December 1, 2017. https://www.timeanddate.com/weather/jamaica/montego-bay/historic?month=10&year=2015.

Rezvany, Roxy. "The Challenges of Running a Queer Homeless Shelter in Jamaica." Vice (New York, New York) March 21, 2016. https://www.vice.com/en_us/article/yvx7bk/the-struggle-for-queer-shelters-in-jamaica.

Ruiz, Alicia, Florina Serbanescu, and Danielle Suchdev. *Reproductive Health Survey: Jamaica, 2008*. Kingston, Jamaica: National Family Planning Board, June 2010. http://jnfpb.org/assets/2008 percent20Final percent20Report percent20Jamaica.pdf.

Scott, James C. *Domination and the Arts of Resistance: Hidden Transcripts*. New Haven: Yale University Press, 1990.

Simpkins, Antwann Michael. "Under Siege: Black Women, the Choreography of Law, and the Public Carceral Sphere." Master's Thesis: University of California, Los Angeles 2016. https://escholarship.org/uc/item/1244f7q6.

Spillers, Hortense. "Interstices: A Small Drama of Words." In *Black, White, and in Color: Essays on American Literature and Culture*, by Hortense J. Spillers, 152–175. Chicago: University of Chicago Press, 2003.

"Weather for NKJS—July, 2013." *Weather Underground* (Ann Arbor, Michigan). Accessed October 22, 2017. https://www.wunderground.com/history/airport/MKJS/2013/7/21/DailyHistory.html?req_city=&req_state=&req_statename=&reqdb.zip=&reqdb.magic=&reqdb.wmo.

White, Chrishana Melissa. "Human Rights and the Impact of Criminalization: Legalizing Homophobia in Jamaica, Nigeria and Uganda." Law School Student Scholarship 325 (2013). http://scholarship.shu.edu/cgi/viewcontent.cgi?article=1325&context=student_scholarship.

Chapter Nine

Traversing Violence

Central American Mujerx *and the Mental Health Impacts of Forced Migration*

Anayeli Marcos, Ana Vidina Hernández, Dora Gonzalez, and Laurie Cook Heffron

Against[1] the enduring backdrop of colonization, civil war, and genocide, increasing flows of individuals and families from the Northern Triangle[2] of Central America (Guatemala, El Salvador, and Honduras) are migrating to the United States as a result of contemporary push factors including gang violence, domestic violence, and other forms of gender-based violence. Particularly, cases of gender-based violence are often under-reported and unrecognized, and governments of these nations have both perpetrated this violence and failed to protect *mujerxs* from it. Notably, the United States' interventionist policies and actions have also contributed to the manifestation of violence. This complex context negatively impacts the health, well-being, and experience of trauma faced by mujerxs who are forced to migrate for their survival. In their transit through Mexico to the United States, forced migrant mujerxs further face violence and exploitation by a host of governmental and criminal networks. Rather than providing comprehensive trauma-informed assistance, Mexico and the United States have responded to forced migration with the punitive measures of detention and deportation.

Substantial growth in migration specifically from the Northern Triangle of Central America to the United States is a recent and growing phenomenon, nearly tripling in number since 1990 (Rosenblum and Brick 2011; Batalova and Lesser 2017). Femicide, governmental tolerance for violence against women, unemployment and underemployment of men, and receiving countries' demand for both domestic labor and sex work are contributing factors to increased internal and international migration, particularly among women in Latin America (Benería, Deere, and Kabeer 2012; Pessar 2005). Furthermore, the Northern Triangle's political and civil conflict of the 1980s, including sexual violence against indigenous communities and internal displacement resulting from internal armed conflict and natural disasters, created an environment ripe for the continued legacy of gender-based violence and proliferation of organized crime (Chazaro, Casey, and Ruhl 2010; Dudley 2012; Paley 2014).

The term gender-based violence (GBV)[3] refers to violence resulting from normative role expectations associated with gender, in addition to gender-related power inequality (Bloom 2008, 14). The United Nations defines GBV as "[An] act of gender-based violence that results in, or is likely to result in, physical, sexual or psychological harm or suffering to women, including threats of such acts, coercion or arbitrary deprivations of liberty, whether occurring in public or in private life" (United Nations 1993, Article 1). It can include physical, sexual, and psychological violence that occurs: in the family; between intimate partners; within the general community; and as violence perpetrated or condoned by the State.

Exposure to GBV in the Northern Triangle ranges from sexual assault and intimate partner violence to femicide, or the killing of women (Menjívar 2011). Recent global data suggests that El Salvador, Honduras, and Guatemala endure the first-, second-, and fourth-highest rates of femicide in the world, respectively (Geneva Declaration 2015). Exposure to gang violence is often gendered and interconnected with women's experiences of intimate partner and sexual violence (Cook Heffron in press). GBV in Central America, however, is shrouded in silence and remains a severely underreported crime due to societal pressures, fear of reprisal, fear of publicity and stigmatization, discriminatory practices by authorities, and low confidence in the justice system (Hume 2004; Hume 2009; United Nations 2004). Given the lack of housing options and insufficient income, it remains difficult for women experiencing abuse to escape violence by relocating within their countries, and migration is often an avenue to escape, seek safety, or resist violence and oppression (Argüelles and Rivero 2004; Salcido and Adelman 2004; Upegui-Hernández 2012; Wagner 2009). The migration process, however, poses further risks of violence, and women are vulnerable to verbal and physical abuse, sexual assault, rape, and other forms of violence on the route through Mexico to the United States (Amnesty International 2010; Infante, Idrovo, Sánchez-Domínguez, Vinhas, and González-Vázquez 2012).

This chapter seeks to explore the social and mental health impacts of GBV as well as the resilience and survival strategies of mujerxs from the Northern Triangle as they travel through Mexico and arrive in the United States These ideas will be explored using a series of brief case sketches[4] compiled from multiple cases we encountered in our work with immigrant women and within immigrant detention centers in Texas through our roles as advocates, social workers, and researchers. First, we introduce Patricia, a Honduran woman who fled her home after the gang-related murder of her son and continued threats of gang violence. Her case highlights migrant survivors' exposure to grief, loss, and cultural bereavement. Next, a snapshot of Sara's experience illustrates the mental health impacts of gender-based violence on immigrant women. Finally, we explore the biopsychosocial impact of immigrant detention on survivors of GBV through the lens of Maria's story. These case sketches offer snapshots we hope will elicit further questions and discussion about the ways that violence, in its various manifestations, is woven throughout Central American mujerxs' migration experiences.

CASE SKETCH—HONDURAS

Patricia is a forty-year-old single mother of two girls aged thirteen and eight. She and her daughters originate from a small canton [district] in Honduras. As her family's sole financial provider, Patricia woke up at the crack of dawn to prepare the tamales and the atole she sold outside her home. Her children's father abandoned his family five years ago. Patricia never remarried; subsequently, she opened her small household business. One ill-fated day, she experienced a great loss—the death of her sixteen-year-old son. In the weeks leading up to his death, a local gang aggressively tried to recruit her son. He refused to join and was later abducted and killed. Despite Patricia's insistence with police to open a homicide investigation, the police refused, fearing gang retaliation. A year after her son's murder, Patricia received an extortion note under her door demanding 25,000 lempiras. She grew anxious and vigilant. She had been seeing gang members walking around her house for a few weeks and worried they would harm her and her daughters. The note said she had three days to gather the money, seal it in an envelope, and leave the envelope in a specific drop box nearby. Patricia did not have the money. Three days passed and Patricia received threatening calls from different men saying they would kill her family or go to the children's school to kidnap the girls. Patricia unplugged her landline but knew it would not end there. On a separate night, she heard voices and movement outside her home. The noise woke up the girls but she urged them to sleep. She feared her family could be killed that night for failing to pay the extortion fee. However, the voices quelled after some time. She lay awake, frightened. When dawn broke, she peered outside her front window, and with no one in sight, she decided to go outside. Freshly painted on the side of her house: three coffins and three skulls. Above the coffins read the word, "muerte" [death]. Patricia had no time to cry before she realized her daughters had followed her; her eight-year-old dropped to the ground, fainting from witnessing the image. At that moment, Patricia decided to flee to the United States with her daughters. Patricia felt she had no other choice; she could not pay. She suspected that this extortion was also retaliation from her earlier attempts to find her son's killers. She fled in the middle of the night.

Grief is a normal, non-pathological experience following bereavement, but prolonged affect may have detrimental effects. Individuals experience loss which produces grief as a multidimensional experience resulting from a significant loss from the death of a loved one, loss of a physical ability, a change in household membership or family boundaries, a fundamental change in one's community, and/or the loss of one's social structure and culture—to name a few (Pomeroy 2011). This experience may involve the emotional, cognitive, physical, social, behavioral, and spiritual components of a person's life. Many of these losses are often devastating and overwhelming and can have lifelong effects, some of which can be traumatic. In turn, these types of losses can lead to chronic mental and physical health problems.

In Patricia's case, the losses she experienced involved the disappearance and death of a loved one and the loss of social structure and culture due to forced migration. Though some of these losses may be universally experienced, Patricia's case—and that of other Central American mujerxs migrants—are pertinent for study, given the rate of homicidal and gender-based violence cases in Honduras, El Salvador, and Guatemala, and the added gendered experience of migration.

Human-generated traumatic events are identified as causing a severe and enduring reaction in survivors. Charuvastra and Cloitre's (2008) systematic study of social bonds and PTSD conceptualized the social ecology of PTSD as highly dependent on social phenomena. The appraisal of an event as human-caused, in particular, appears in PTSD studies as particularly fear-inducing (303). Traumas of a non-personal nature (i.e., "accident" or "natural disaster with fire" or witnessing a trauma) have conditional probabilities for PTSD whereas violence by rape, combat exposure, childhood neglect, and physical abuse, assault, and being threatened with a weapon are among traumas associated with a high rate of PTSD. Interpersonal traumas, lack of social support—an effective emotional regulator—and social bonds—particularly between caregivers and children—influence how children respond to traumatic events and modulate feelings of fear versus those of safety (302). Evidence from neurochemistry and neurobiology further explains how social phenomena modulate the fear circuitry in the brain, and suggests that social experience can shape and alter the brain's behavior and chemistry in the context of traumatic stress (302).

When loss and grief caused by human-designed violence is considered, "the sense that death is 'untimely,' 'unfair,' and 'unnatural' intensifies feelings of shock, loss, disbelief, and anger" (Aldrich and Kallivayalil 2016, 25). Homicide is one particular type of death that could be understood by parameters of "untimely," "unfair," loss and anger. Although research suggests social support can buffer and mitigate the impact of traumatic events, an individual's assumptive view of safety may be altered completely. An individual may experience the context they live in as having new attributes: fear, vigilance, vulnerability, yearning, consuming revenge fantasies, powerlessness, and so on. (26). This change can make it difficult for survivors to seek support from their social networks because of distrust; a sense of self characterized by vulnerability, shame, or damage; or because personal grieving becomes culturally unacceptable after a specific period of time and leads to isolation (Armour 2002; Charuvastra and Cloitre 2008; Herman 1992; Horowitz 1986; Aldrich and Kallivayalil 2016, 26).

The duration and expression of loss can vary by culture. Individuals may keep codes and lengths of culturally acceptable mourning processes about bereavement. However, when grief lasts beyond the culturally accepted period of mourning, the open expression of grief may be sanctioned. When the grief process worsens and endures, grief may be considered abnormal and maladaptive, and associated with an individual's inability to process the bereavement in a healthy manner, suggesting a chronic grief pattern. When individuals experience a chronic grief pattern it may further devolve into Complicated Grief Disorder—a frozen or stuck state of chronic mourning with psychological protest against recognizing the loss, and reluctance to make adaptations around the absence (Hollander 2016, 294). Without this understanding, cultural sanctioning around bereavement can be harmful for an individual experiencing prolonged grief. This could lead into a different layering of grief called disenfranchised grief. This theoretical phenomenon describes a societal and individual response to grief and loss that inherently denies recognition, legitimization, or support of the loss or grief being experienced by an individual (Hollander 2016, 295). Survivors may often choose to omit pieces of their personal narratives. The cost of connection to others may be at the expense of their authenticity. Other dimensions of withdrawing and feeling apart may include relentless rumination of the details of the murder and loved one's last minutes (Aldrich and Kallivayalil 2016, 27).

In his qualitative fieldwork with parents of missing persons in Uganda, Theo Hollander (2016) examines the emotional, social, cultural, and socioeconomic aspects of the ambiguity that relatives of missing persons experience in the aftermath of wartime disappearances. This article's theoretical framework around "ambiguous loss" helps frame forced disappearances and/or unresolved murder cases in context as is pertinent in this case study. Boss describes two types of ambiguous loss: (1) a situation in which a person is physically absent but psychologically present in the minds of friends and relatives; and (2) a situation in which a person is physically present but psychologically absent (295). In both, loss causes a range of stressors that freeze the grief process and prevent healthy processing. Boss (2006) classifies ambiguous loss as the most stressful and traumatizing loss since there is no verification, no closure, no rituals for support, and thus no resolution of grief (144). Relatedly, Patricia may have experienced the immediate physical but perhaps not psychological loss of her son with his abduction until the confirmation of his death—an ambiguous loss.

Due to forced migration, Patricia is also susceptible to grief reaction from the loss of social structure and culture. Eisenbruch (1991) describes this loss as the loss of the familiar, including language (colloquial and dialect), attitudes, values, social structures, and support networks. Social structural and cultural loss is a consequence of relocation and migration. Grieving from this loss can be viewed as a normal reaction; however, if the symptoms cause significant distress or impairment and last for a specified period of time, psychiatric intervention may be warranted. Forced migration because of an ongoing threat of violence—threat of death, extortion, kidnapping, sexual violence, community violence—is inherently damaging because of the involuntarily nature. Eisenbruch (1991) defines this type of grief as cultural bereavement:

> The experience of the uprooted person—or group—resulting from loss of social structures, cultural values and self-identity: the person—or group—continues to live in the past, is visited by supernatural forces from the past while asleep or awake, suffers feelings of guilt over abandoning culture and homeland, feels pain if memories of the past begin to fade, but finds constant images of the past (including traumatic images) intruding into daily life, yearns to complete obligations to the dead, and feels stricken by anxieties, morbid thoughts, and anger that mar the ability to get on with daily life. (Sec. "Cultural Bereavement")

Acculturation and potential discrepancy between attainment of goals and actual achievement are pieces of social structure and culture loss faced in latter stages of the migration process. Migrants come into contact with the "majority" or "dominant" culture in voluntary and involuntary ways. Social adjustment considers the duration of relocation; the similarity or dissimilarity between the culture of origin and the culture of settlement; language and social support systems; acceptance by the "majority" culture; access and acceptance by the migrant community in the host country; employment; and housing (Bhugra and Becker 2005, 21). On a personal level, an individual may experience a sense of rejection, alienation, and poor self-esteem if they feel isolated from their culture, unaccepted by the "majority culture," and lacking in social support (21). An individual may experience a loss of cultural identity as they experience de-culturation during the assimilation process as they move within the host society. Psychosocial changes may incur from acculturation, a process that may be voluntary or forced, in the contact between divergent values, customs, beliefs, and language (21). These biological, psychological, and social variables may then heavily influence an individual's capacity to grieve and adapt.

CASE SKETCH—EL SALVADOR

Sara, thirty-eight, was held at a Texas immigrant family detention center for several days with her five-year-old son and three-year-old daughter. She had been at the center for about five days and had arrived in the United States ten days earlier. Her credible fear interview, which would determine whether or not she could be released from the center to seek asylum, was scheduled in three days.

In her home country, Sara lived with her husband and two children in El Salvador. When she first met her husband, he treated her well and was kind to her. Once they were living together and she was pregnant with their first child, he began to drink heavily and would come home on weekends and hit her. One night he hit her so violently that she had to be taken to the hospital and had a miscarriage. Later she became pregnant two more times and gave birth to a boy and a girl.

Throughout the eleven years of their marriage, her husband was frequently physically abusive, and he was also occasionally sexually abusive. He often came home late and demanded that she make him a hot meal. If she refused, he threw hot food or plates at her. He often accused her of cheating on him with other men, and he frequently stayed with other women and sent Sara pictures of these encounters. He controlled the amount of money she could spend and rarely let her leave the house. He insulted her, saying that women were "dogs" and that he didn't care what happened to her or their daughter—only what happened to their son. Even so, he continuously threatened to find her and kill her if she ever left with the children.

The violence from her husband escalated in the summer of 2017, particularly as he began seeing another woman. She began to plan how she would leave, knowing that it would need to be when he was not at the house. Toward the end of that summer, members of a regional gang came to her children's school and made kidnapping threats. Fearing for their safety, Sara put their plan into action and left her home with her two children. She fled to her mother's home for one night and then left the country. She made it to the United States with her two children, crossing the Mexico border, and was detained in a hielera, a perrera[5]*, and ultimately an immigrant family detention center in Texas. While speaking with a social worker, Sara also revealed that she witnessed domestic violence as a child between her own parents and experienced physical and emotional abuse from her father.*

Sara's case is representative of many mujerxs who flee Central American countries with their children to seek asylum. She experienced multilayered violence, including societal maintenance of unequal gender norms, the pervasiveness of gang violence, and continued domestic violence over more than a decade of her life. In these situations, her position in society as a woman greatly impacted her experience of abuse. Her story helps us understand the context of gender-based violence and how cycles of power and control lead to the traumatization of mujerxs in these situations.

Madrigal and Tejeda (2009) discuss the importance of considering the historical and political context of El Salvador when discussing GBV. This includes the impacts of the twelve-year war, which lasted from 1980 to 1992 and left 75,000 dead, over 350,000 wounded, tens of thousands tortured or abducted, and around five million displaced (Ching, 2016). It also includes economic and social instability, and increased gang violence. Specifically, "from 2001–2004, approximately 2900 women were murdered" (Romeva I Rueda 2007, 14). Hume (2008) similarly references the civil war and its impact on the complexity of violence in El Salvador that includes direct state control and symbolic violence that normalizes inequality. One of the ways this occurs is through the view that domestic violence is a *private matter*. Mujerxs often state that in trying to report to the police, they were told that this was a private family matter that police would not interfere with. Furthermore, the climate of fear created by the increasing gang violence and control in El Salvador contributes to the normalization of violent acts in society. As in the case of Sara, it also creates additional reasons for mujerxs to face violence and to flee.

Research on GBV confirms that mujerxs are more likely to face violence from men that they know, rather than from strangers (Hume 2008; Perez and Johnson 2008). A 2008 governmental survey in El Salvador revealed that nearly one half of mujerxs nationwide had experienced violence at the hands of their partner while in a relationship (Amnesty International 2014). Madrigal and Tejeda (2009) analyze GBV as including the two primary factors of violent expressions of masculinity and unequal gender relations. They further discuss the ways in which "the environment, socialization, and culturally dominant ideas and beliefs regarding acceptable masculine behavior" shape the ways violence is expressed by men in El Salvador (369). Hume (2008) argues that gender inequality and male privilege affect how notions of violence are "constructed, internalized, and reproduced" (62). Furthermore, the ways in which violence, particularly in the family unit, becomes normalized can impact how individuals perceive and define what constitutes violent acts.

Survivors of domestic and sexual violence often experience a sense of hopelessness and isolation as they attempt to cope with the traumatic events they have gone through. Hopelessness can be seen as feelings of despair and not seeing a way out, which can evoke a lack of internal and external autonomy and control over one's life. This can keep individuals from making life-changing decisions due to a decrease in confidence in believing that one can escape and change their current situation. Feelings of isolation can increase physical and emotional detachment from others (Karakurt, Smith, & Whiting, 2014).

Power and control, based on both structural and gender inequality, are viewed as key components of domestic violence (Grose and Grabe 2014; Anderson 1997). Lehmann, Simmons, and Pillai (2012) discuss the concept of coercive controlling violence through a study with the Checklist of Controlling Behaviors (CCB), which acknowledges both physical and emotional violence as part of control and coercion. For the purposes of their study, the authors described coercion as force or threats, while they described control as being structural and including the creation of barriers to resources and personal freedom. Of the ten subscales on the CCB, Sara described experiencing all: physical abuse, sexual abuse, emotional abuse, economic abuse, intimidation, threats, minimizing and denying, blaming, isolation, and male privilege (Lehmann, Simmons, and Pillai 2012).

Grose and Grabe (2014) describe power as "having both the capacity and the opportunity to fulfill or impede personal and relational needs" (975). They discuss the two processes of "individual power to" (the ability to achieve self-fulfillment regarding personal goals and behaviors without affecting others' opportunities) and "interpersonal power over" (one's ability to control, manipulate, or win a conflict with others). In the case of Sara, she lived in an extremely unequal relationship with her husband in terms of power and control. She had limited "individual power to," in that she did not have many opportunities to fulfill her own goals because of societal pressures and her husband's control over her life. Her husband held a great deal of "interpersonal power over," as he controlled her financial access, physical movement, sexual health, domestic work, and child rearing. Inequality in decision making in particular has been shown to be a primary factor in rates of violence against mujerxs (978). When placed in the context of a community largely controlled by gangs with a history of civil war and state abuse of power, Sara faced gender-based oppression from many areas of her life.

In this chapter we draw on Supin's (2016) definition of trauma as "an experience, or pattern of experiences, that impairs the proper functioning of the person's stress-response system, making it more reactive or sensitive" (5). Bruce Perry, MD, PhD, also discusses the way in which fear shuts down the reasoning part of the brain and makes individuals more compliant toward authority. Perry further adds that hunger, thirst, and exhaustion have a similar effect—thus impacting poorer individuals more (13). An individual who faces this type of experience consistently over time may live in a constant state of fear and develop PTSD (Post Traumatic Stress Disorder) symptoms. Salcioglu, Urhan, Pirinccioglu, and Aydin (2017) note that survivors feel distress and a lack of control over stressful events, in addition to being fearful of reliving the same domestic violence events and fearing for their lives.

The connection between domestic violence and PTSD is important to consider when discussing the mental health impacts for Central American mujerxs who leave abusive relationships and migrate to the United States Symptoms of PTSD, depression, and anxiety are common among survivors of domestic violence (Salcioglu, Urhan, Pirinccioglu, and Aydin 2017; Perez and Johnson 2008; Jones, Hughes, and Unterstaller 2001). Central American immigrants in particular have a high prevalence of PTSD from childhood experiences and community, political, drug gang, and interpersonal violence (Kaltman, Hurtado de Mendoza, Gonzales, Serrano, and Guarnaccia 2011). Another challenge facing these mujerxs is often a lack of community support when attempting to leave violent situations.

Considering the impacts of childhood trauma for victims of domestic violence takes into account compounded trauma experiences over time. Childhood trauma can be a risk factor for interpersonal violence (IPV) and IPV can exacerbate PTSD symptoms from traumatic childhood experiences (Gobin, Iverson, Mitchell, Vaughn, and Resick 2013; Jones, Hughes, and Unterstaller 2001). In the case of Sara, the childhood violence she experienced may have contributed to the PTSD symptoms she experienced after surviving domestic violence in her own adult relationship. This also creates implications for Sara's two children—namely, how will the domestic violence they witnessed and the intergenerational transmission of trauma impact their future mental health? Studies indicate that children of women who have been victims of sexual assault are more likely to also become victims of abuse when they get older (Wearick-Silva et al. 2014). McFarlane et al. (2014) also found that, "[A]s abused women's behavioral functioning problems increase there is an increase in behavioral problems in their children," which could lead to various internalized and externalized behaviors affecting emotional expression, psychological well-being, and overall development (2240). Immigrant women were also at higher risk of negative mental health outcomes for both mother and child due to the heightened stress of being undocumented or living with precarious legal status (McFarlane et al. 2014). Violence against mujerxs is often normalized in many Central American countries, which makes it harder for women and their families to address this cycle of trauma and keep it from being transmitted to other family members and loved ones.

CASE SKETCH—GUATEMALA

Maria is a twenty-two-year-old woman from Guatemala who was recently transferred to the Karnes Detention Center with her one-year-old daughter. Maria had been at the center for three days and had arrived in the United States approximately a week earlier. She was awaiting to appear before an asylum officer in order to see if she had a credible fear claim which, if granted, would allow her to continue pursuing her immigration case from outside of the detention center.

Before arriving in the United States, Maria had lived with her husband and his family in Guatemala. Maria became pregnant and did not foresee what would happen to her later on after her daughter was born. Maria began to notice that her husband would drink a lot and would often come home late at night intoxicated. She also began to suspect that her husband was having an affair with another woman but did not know how to address this conversation. Her husband became more violent and would hit her whenever Maria "did something wrong." His parents did not step in whenever Maria got hit, and she decided to report this to local law enforcement.

Maria noticed the birth of her daughter did not do anything to help alleviate the marital problems she and her husband were having. Maria confronted her husband and stated that she wanted to get a divorce and again her husband hit her and yelled at her, stating that she was useless and no good for him. Maria went to the police again to report the incident and filed a restraining order and a petition for child support. She was granted the restraining order for three months, but Maria began receiving threats from her husband's new partner.

Soon enough Maria found herself being kicked out of her husband's parents' home, and she became homeless. Despite moving away, Maria still received threats over the phone, and she decided to come to the United States to seek asylum. Since being inside the detention center Maria has received little to no guidance from officers in how to file forms, petitions, or request legal assistance. She is no longer called by her name, but by an A-Number,[6] *and her visits and mail are always monitored. She is also concerned about her daughter growing up within the walls of a detention center, where she has little control over how her case will be handled.*

Maria's story provides an example of the difficulties mujerxs face in their home countries, and—especially in Guatemala—reports of women being killed through sexual and domestic violence are a national concern for advocates seeking to reduce GBV. Violence against women continues to be a pervasive problem in Guatemala, in part due to "[a] culture that devalues and subordinates women, as manifested by anachronistic criminal laws and gender-based discrimination in the home and workplace" in addition to the "widespread impunity for crimes against women that traces from the country's thirty-six-year civil war" (Reimann 2009, 1200). As a consequence of this history, mujerxs do not feel safe and comfortable reporting crimes to authorities, as illustrated in Maria's case.

These experiences of violence can also be perpetuated during the migration journey, as mujerxs leave their countries for various reasons. In the migration journey, mujerxs become victims of traumatic experiences including rape, sexual assault, kidnapping, extortion, trafficking, and so much more.

The journey itself is often long and exhausting, making it difficult for the body to regulate at a healthy and functional capacity. From boarding trains, to walking long distances, to spending the night at shelters or in the streets, these mujerxs physically, emotionally, and psychologically endure multiple experiences that can heighten mental health concerns.

Mujerxs making their way to the United States often spend some time in Mexico in the hope of finding assistance and help. Mexico, as a response to the increase in Central American migrants arriving at its borders, has tightened security and increased deportations. Lopez and Hastings (2016) found that, "In 2015, the Mexican government deported 190,366 people. Of those deported 150,170 were from the NTCA, including 70,493 Guatemalans, 50,527 Hondurans, and 29,150 Salvadorans" (1107). In addition to their analysis, Lopez and Hastings report "An estimated 60% of women suffered rape during their journey through Mexico; while some current reports estimate that this statistic has increased to 80% of migrant women" (1116). Mujerxs who identify as indigenous are even more vulnerable to facing discrimination and allocating services due to "language barriers and illiteracy" that "further increase the likelihood that indigenous women will be victimized and concurrently decrease their ability to seek protection and redress" (1117).

Once migrating to Mexico, many mujerxs realize the government does not provide enough protection or assistance in order to make them feel safe and secure. Despite Mexico receiving many asylum applications each year and having established progressive humanitarian laws and policies, in 2016 Mexico only granted asylum to about 21% of applicants. This low acceptance rate may be a sign that Mexico faces its own dilemmas in finding solutions to the growing crisis facing Central American immigrants as they make their way to their borders. In addition, many Central American migrants in Mexico are not aware of their right to seek asylum even though they have a credible case that could be granted. Lopez and Hastings (2016) found that "68% of people in Mexico's largest detention center, Siglo XXI Immigration Station in Tapachula, were unaware of their right to seek asylum" through a report written by the Inter-American Commission in 2013 (1119). Despite the hopes mujerxs have in seeking better treatment in the United States, sadly the reality could not be any different as they face another oppressive structural system that criminalizes their experiences in detention.

DETENTION IN THE UNITED STATES

When asylum-seeking migrants arrive at the U.S. border, many are apprehended, processed, and detained by border enforcement agencies. This is disconcerting given that prolonged detention appears to contribute substantially to the risk of depression, PTSD, and other mental health outcomes in refugees and asylum seekers. Keller et al. (2003) studied asylum seekers detained in the metropolitan New York area, finding high rates of psychological distress. This study identified 77% of participants presented clinically significant symptoms of anxiety, 86% had depression, and 50% had PTSD, and symptom severity was significantly correlated with the length of time individuals had been detained (2). Follow-up interviews conducted two months later revealed marked decreases in distress among those who had been released from detention (granted asylum) but a worsening of symptoms among those still detained (2–3). As the studies show, migrant detention is a harmful and traumatizing experience.

Furthermore, detention includes a process of grief and loss for migrant families as detainees are often placed in centers far away from where they live and work, and are *physically* moved quickly across towns, cities, and state lines (Mountz 2012). Once inside these facilities, detainees are stripped of various forms of autonomy/control including: their names (often called out by the number assigned to them), what they wear, what they eat, where they go, and someone even monitors their mail, visitations, and phone calls. These limits on basic needs and interactions can cause detainees to not feel safe, make them unwilling to express feelings or emotions, increase isolation, increase stress and anxiety, and overall pose a risk factor for mental health concerns.

In addition, Tania Storm and Marianne Engberg (2013) further highlight the lack of compliance and accountability detention centers have in upholding policies that help detainees. There have been reports of sexual assault, harassment, suicide attempts, denial of medical help, and even deaths inside detention centers across the United States. For individuals who have not committed a serious crime besides crossing a border, these detainees are treated as criminals and are often placed in questionable living conditions that put their lives and their mental well-being in danger.

DISCUSSION

In sum, violence both impacts migration and is impacted by migration, and in turn incurs great medical, emotional, legal, and financial costs for individual women, their families, and the U.S. and Central American societies at large. Patricia, Sara, and Maria's cases highlight the multiple mental health concerns women carry with them when migrating to the United States. Given premigration trauma and abuse, as well as violence endured during migration, mujerxs experience grief, loss, cultural bereavement, depression, and PTSD.

These experiences are often exacerbated by immigrant detention. Given the costs of these intersections of migration and violence, coupled with the numbers of Central American women crossing the border into the United States and the increasing criminalization of asylum-seekers, it is crucial that advocates, practitioners, and policymakers recognize and address survivors' needs.

For those released from detention and permitted to stay in the United States to seek asylum, mental health implications of previous trauma and of detention must be addressed after release. Criminalization, precarious legal status, financial insecurity, and family separation continue to trouble asylum-seekers after detention. It is crucial that social service and mental health providers gain a better understanding of the migration experience and detention center conditions in order to best serve this population as they leave detention and enter the United States as undocumented women needing legal and social support. Social service providers should also adopt a trauma-informed approach when providing services and referrals to previously detained women. It is equally important that service providers engage in Know Your Rights workshops to provide immigrants with vital information regarding immigration laws.

Not all women in detention pass the credible or reasonable fear interviews and continue with an asylum application. Those who are not released into the United States are deported to their country of origin, incurring implications for the women and for service providers in Central America. For those who have been through potentially traumatic experiences in their home countries, during their migration, and in detention, being deported may add an additional level of fear and stress as they are returned to the situations that they fled. Considering the implications for mental health, whether or not they face further threats from gangs or former partners, mujerxs are often living in precarious situations with a lack of resources. Systems should be put in place to help women prepare for deportation and address potential safety and security risks. For social service providers in Central America, taking into consideration the unique needs of individuals deported from the United States and providing services accordingly will be important to address their circumstances.

The Trump Administration's reversal of Temporary Protected Status (TPS), a program that provides temporary lawful status and work authorization to immigrants from countries affected by armed conflict, natural disasters, or other strife, has been one of the most consequential to date. With Homeland Security ending the humanitarian program for El Salvador and Nicaragua, Salvadorans and Nicaraguans living and working in the United States for over a decade are now ordered to leave the country ("Secretary of Homeland . . . El Salvador" 2018; "Acting Secretary . . . Nicaragua and Honduras" 2017). In addition, it is also predicted others in the programs may soon lose protections, namely Hondurans. With this recent change, hundreds of thousands of families—Salvadorans being the largest group to benefit from

TPS, with close to 200,000 recipients—are in jeopardy of losing their livelihood (Jordan 2018). Families with mixed legal statuses are in danger of being forcibly separated. Many parents and/or legal guardians will be forced to decide between returning to El Salvador with their children, needing to rebuild and facing safety threats, leaving them with guardians in the United States, or remaining in the country at the risk of arrest and deportation (Jordan 2018).

Despite the many barriers mujerxs from Central America face in seeking safety and protection, we cannot overlook the incredible strengths that women have in succeeding and enduring such hardships. Through the facilitation of a support group with detained women at the T. Don Hutto Detention Center in Texas, we have been able to see the success that such programs and group interventions can have in the overall well-being of women who have gone through traumatic experiences. This support group is facilitated through volunteers of the YWCA of Austin, who receive specialized training and clinical supervision in bringing emotional and psychological support to detained women. In this support group, facilitators and detained women are able to discuss difficult topics ranging from sexual assault, grief, and loss, to the experiences of being in detention and going through the asylum process.

CONCLUSION

It will remain difficult to assess the breadth and depth of violence experienced by Central American migrant women as long as the lack of legal immigration status in the United States keeps women in the shadows. It is imperative that this contemporary context generates deep and critical discussions of policy discourses and developments, including those related to the detention of women fleeing violence. If migrant women describe abusive relationships, assault during migration, and/or further victimization upon arrival in the United States, we must remain both vigilant and diligent in how we make sense of that in our responses. In particular, when most legal, policy, and social service strategies are targeted at one instance of violence or one relationship and are categorized as mutually exclusive (rape or domestic violence or gang violence), are these responses capable of fully addressing the experiences of migrant women? These conversations must take place at the community, statewide, and national levels and must preserve the voices and solutions of migrant women themselves.

NOTES

1. We use the term *mujerxs* to reflect and acknowledge a more fluid notion of gender.

2. The term "Northern Triangle" is frequently used in research to demarcate the region composed of Honduras, El Salvador, and Guatemala though its use is problematic due to its historically militaristic and imperialistic origin.

3. While gender-based violence impacts individuals across multiple gender identities, we will focus on the manifestations of GBV among Central American migrant women.

4. Each case presented in this chapter represents a de-identified, reconstructed case sketch. Case sketches were compiled of components of multiple cases encountered by the authors in our direct social work practice with asylum-seeking women and in immigrant detention centers in Texas. They represent fictionalized composites of real cases and were developed for the purpose of illustrating the themes included in this chapter. Names associated with each case sketch are pseudonyms. The development of these case sketches was also informed by original research (see Cook Heffron in press) and the existing empirical literature.

5. *Hieleras* and *perreras* are short-term immigrant detention facilities operated by U.S. Customs & Border Protection. *Hieleras*, "freezers" or "ice boxes," incurred this moniker due to their consistently low temperatures. After spending time in a *hielera*, immigrants are sometimes transferred to another form of temporary detention, a *perrera*, referring to these facilities' resemblance to dog kennels.

6. An A-Number is known as an Alien Registration Number that is composed of an eight- or nine-digit number that is assigned to a noncitizen of the United States.

WORKS CITED

Aldrich, Holly, and Diya Kallivayalil. 2016. "Traumatic Grief After Homicide: Intersections of Individual and Community Loss." *Illness, Crisis & Loss* 24 (1): 15–33. https://doi.org/10.1177/1054137315587630.

Amnesty International. 2010. "Invisible Victims: Migrants on the Move in Mexico." London: Amnesty International Publications. https://www.amnestyusa.org/reports/invisible-victims-migrants-on-the-move-in-mexico/.

———. 2014. "On the Brink of Death: Violence Against Women and the Abortion Ban in El Salvador." Peter Benenson House. https://www.amnestyusa.org/files/el_salvador_report_-_on_the_brink_of_death.pdf.

Anderson, Kristin L. 1997. "Gender, Status, and Domestic Violence: An Integration of Feminist and Family Violence Approaches." *Journal of Marriage and Family* 59 (3): 655–69. https://doi.org/10.2307/353952.

Argüelles, Lourdes, and Anne M. Rivero. 1993. "Gender/Sexual Orientation Violence And Transnational Migration: Conversations with Some Latinas We Think We Know." *Urban Anthropology and Studies of Cultural Systems and World Economic Development* 22 (3/4): 259–75.

Armour, Marilyn. 2002. "Experiences of Covictims of Homicide: Implications for Research and Practice." *Trauma, Violence, & Abuse* 3 (2): 109–24. https://doi.org/10.1177/15248380020032002.

Ayón, Cecilia, Jill T. Messing, Maria Gurrola, and Dellanira Valencia-Garcia. 2017. "The Oppression of Latina Mothers: Experiences of Exploitation, Violence, Marginalization, Cultural Imperialism, and Powerlessness in Their Everyday Lives." *Violence Against Women*, October, 1077801217724451. https://doi.org/10.1177/1077801217724451.

Batalova, Jeanne, and Gabriel Lesser. 2017. "Central American Immigrants in the United States." Migrationpolicy.org. April 4, 2017. https://www.migrationpolicy.org/article/central-american-immigrants-united-states.

Benería, Lourdes, Carmen Diana Deere, and Naila Kabeer. 2012. "Gender and International Migration: Globalization, Development, and Governance." *Feminist Economics* 18 (2): 1–33. https://doi.org/10.1080/13545701.2012.688998.

Bhugra, Dinesh, and Matthew Becker. 2005. "Migration, Cultural Bereavement and Cultural Identity." *World Psychiatry* 4 (1): 18–24.

Boss, Pauline. 2006. *Loss, Trauma, and Resilience: Therapeutic Work with Ambiguous Loss*. New York, NY: Norton.

Charuvastra, Anthony, and Marylene Cloitre. 2008. "Social Bonds and Posttraumatic Stress Disorder." *Annual Review of Psychology* 59: 301–28. https://doi.org/10.1146/annurev.psych.58.110405.085650.

Cházaro, Angélica. 2010. "Getting Away with Murder: Guatemala's Failure to Protect Women and Rodi Alvarado's Quest for Safety." EIGE. 2010. http://eige.europa.eu/rdc/library/resource/IAV_ADL229835.

Ching, E. K. (2016). *Stories of civil war in el salvador: A battle over memory*. Chapel Hill: The University of North Carolina Press.

Cook Heffron, Laurie. (in press). "'Salía de Uno Y Me Metí En Otro:' Exploring the Migration-Violence Nexus among Central American Women." *Violence Against Women*.

Daley, Dawn. 2014. *Drug War Capitalism*. Oakland, CA: AK Press.

Department of Homeland Security. 2017. "Acting Secretary of Homeland Security Kirstjen M. Nielsen Announcement on Temporary Protected Status for Nicaragua and Honduras." https://www.dhs.gov/news/2018/01/08/secretary-homeland-security-kirstjen-m-nielsen-announcement-temporary-protected.

———. 2018. "Secretary of Homeland Security Kirstjen M. Nielsen Announcement on Temporary Protected Status for El Salvador." https://www.dhs.gov/news/2018/01/08/secretary-homeland-security-kirstjen-m-nielsen-announcement-temporary-protected.

Diaz, Gabriela, and Gretchen Kuhner. 2007. "Women Migrants in Transit and Detention in Mexico." Migrationpolicy.org. https://www.migrationpolicy.org/article/women-migrants-transit-and-detention-mexico.

Diaz, Gabriela, and Sarah Gammage. 2016. "Aiding Central America's 'Women on the Run.'" NACLA. 2016. /news/2016/01/06/aiding-central-america-women-run.

Dominguez, Silvia, and Cecilia Menjivar. 2014. "Beyond Individual and Visible Acts of Violence: A Framework to Examine the Lives of Women in Low-Income Neighborhoods." *Women's Studies International Forum* 44 (May): 184–95. https://doi.org/10.1016/j.wsif.2014.01.012.

Dudley, Steven. 2012. "Transnational Crime in Mexico and Central America: Its Evolution and Role in International Migration." Migrationpolicy.org. 2012. https://www.migrationpolicy.org/research/RMSG-CentAm-transnational-crime.

Eguizábal, Cristina, Karise Curtis, Matthew Ingram, Aaron Korthuis, and Eric Olson.
———. 2014. "Crime and Violence in Central America's Northern Triangle: How U.S. Policy Responses Are Helping, Hurting, and Can Be Improved." Wilson Center. 2014. https://www.wilsoncenter.org/publication/crime-and-violence-central-americas-northern-triangle-how-us-policy-responses-are.

Eisenbruch, Maurice. 1991. "From Post-Traumatic Stress Disorder to Cultural Bereavement: Diagnosis of Southeast Asian Refugees." *Social Science & Medicine (1982)* 33 (6): 673–80.

Ellsberg, Mary. 2006. "Violence against Women and the Millennium Development Goals: Facilitating Women's Access to Support." *International Journal of Gynecology & Obstetrics*, World Report on Women's Health 2006; Women's Right to Health and the Millenium Development Goals; Promoting Partnerships to Improve Access, 94 (3): 325–32. https://doi.org/10.1016/j.ijgo.2006.04.021.

Ellsberg, Mary, Henrica AFM Jansen, Lori Heise, Charlotte H. Watts, and Claudia Garcia-Moreno. 2008. "Intimate Partner Violence and Women's Physical and Mental Health in the WHO Multi-Country Study on Women's Health and Domestic Violence: An Observational Study." *The Lancet* 371 (9619): 1165–72. https://doi.org/10.1016/S0140-6736(08)60522-X.

Garcia-Moreno, Claudia, Lori Heise, Henrica Jansen, Mary Ellsberg, and Charlotte Watts. 2005. "Public Health. Violence against Women." *Science* (New York, NY) 310 (5752): 1282–83. https://doi.org/10.1126/science.1121400.

Geneva Declaration (2015). "Global burden of armed violence 2015: Every body counts." Retrieved from http://www.genevadeclaration.org/measurability/global-burden-of-armed-violence/global-burden-of-armed-violence-2015.html.

Gobin, Robyn L., Katherine M. Iverson, Karen Mitchell, Rachel Vaughn, and Patricia A. Resick. 2013. "The Impact of Childhood Maltreatment on PTSD Symptoms among Female Survivors of Intimate Partner Violence." *Violence and Victims* 28 (6): 984–99.

Grose, Rose Grace, and Shelly Grabe. 2014. "The Explanatory Role of Relationship Power and Control in Domestic Violence against Women in Nicaragua: A Feminist Psychology Analysis." *Violence Against Women* 20 (8): 972–93. https://doi.org/10.1177/1077801214546231.

Herman, Judith. 1992. *Trauma and Recovery*. New York, NY: Basic Books.

Hollander, Theo. 2016. "Ambiguous Loss and Complicated Grief: Understanding the Grief of Parents of the Disappeared in Northern Uganda." *Journal of Family Theory & Review* 8 (3): 294–307. https://doi.org/10.1111/jftr.12153.

Horowitz, Mardi Jon. 1986. "Stress-Response Syndromes: A Review of Posttraumatic and Adjustment Disorders." *Hospital & Community Psychiatry* 37 (3): 241–49.

Hume, M. 2008. "The Myths of Violence: Gender, Conflict, and Community in El Salvador." *Latin American Perspectives* 35 (5): 59–76. https://doi.org/10.1177/0094582X08321957.

Hume, Mo. 2004. "'It's as If You Don't Know, Because You Don't Do Anything about It': Gender and Violence in El Salvador." *Environment and Urbanization* 16 (2): 63–72. https://doi.org/10.1177/095624780401600223.

———. 2009. "Researching the Gendered Silences of Violence in El Salvador." *IDS Bulletin* 40 (3): 78–85. https://doi.org/10.1111/j.1759-5436.2009.00042.x.

Infante, César, Alvaro J. Idrovo, Mario S. Sánchez-Domínguez, Stéphane Vinhas, and Tonatiuh González-Vázquez. 2012. "Violence Committed against Migrants in Transit: Experiences on the Northern Mexican Border." *Journal of Immigrant and Minority Health* 14 (3): 449–59. https://doi.org/10.1007/s10903-011-9489-y.

Jones, Loring, Margaret Hughes, and Ulrike Unterstaller. 2001. "Post-Traumatic Stress Disorder (PTSD) in Victims of Domestic Violence: A Review of the Research." *Trauma, Violence, & Abuse* 2 (2): 99–119. https://doi.org/10.1177/1524838001002002001.

Jordan, Miriam. 2018. "Trump Administration Says That Nearly 200,000 Salvadorans Must Leave." *New York Times*, 2018, sec. U.S. https://www.nytimes.com/2018/01/08/us/salvadorans-tps-end.html.

Kaltman, Stacey, Alejandra Hurtado de Mendoza, Felisa A. Gonzales, Adriana Serrano, and Peter J. Guarnaccia. 2011. "Contextualizing the Trauma Experience of Women Immigrants from Central America, South America, and Mexico." *Journal of Traumatic Stress* 24 (6): 635–42. https://doi.org/10.1002/jts.20698.

Karakurt, G., Smith, D., & Whiting, J. (2014). Impact of intimate partner violence on women's mental health. *Journal of Family Violence* 29 (7), 693. 10.1007/s10896-014-9633-2.

Keller, Allen S., Barry Rosenfeld, Chau Trinh-Shevrin, Chris Meserve, Emily Sachs, Jonathan A. Leviss, Elizabeth Singer, et al. 2003. "Mental Health of Detained Asylum Seekers." *Lancet (London, England)* 362 (9397): 1721–23. https://doi.org/10.1016/S0140-6736(03)14846-5.

Lehmann, Peter, Catherine A. Simmons, and Vijayan K. Pillai. 2012. "The Validation of the Checklist of Controlling Behaviors (CCB): Assessing Coercive Control in Abusive Relationships." *Violence Against Women* 18 (8): 913–33. https://doi.org/10.1177/1077801212456522.

Lopez, Esmeralda and Melissa Hastings. 2016. "Overlooked and Unprotected: Central American Indigenous Migrant Women in Mexico." *New York University Journal of International Law and Politics* 48 (4), 1105–24.

Loyd, Jenna, Matt Mitchelson, and Andrew Burridge, eds. 2012. *Beyond Walls and Cages: Prisons, Borders, and Global Crisis*. University of Georgia Press. http://www.jstor.org/stable/j.ctt46njgc.

Madrigal, Larry J., and Walberto V. Tejeda. 2009. "Facing Gender-Based Violence in El Salvador: Contributions from the Social Psychology of Ignacio Martín-Baró." *Feminism & Psychology* 19 (3): 368–74. https://doi.org/10.1177/0959353509105627.

Mares, Sarah, Louise Newman, Michael Dudley, and Fran Gale. 2002. "Seeking Refuge, Losing Hope: Parents and Children in Immigration Detention." *Australasian Psychiatry* 10 (2): 91–96. https://doi.org/10.1046/j.1440-1665.2002.00414.x.

McFarlane, Judith, Lene Symes, Brenda K. Binder, John Maddoux, and Rene Paulson.

———. 2014. "Maternal-Child Dyads of Functioning: The Intergenerational Impact of Violence Against Women on Children." *Maternal and Child Health Journal* 18 (9): 2236–43. https://doi.org/10.1007/s10995-014-1473-4.

Menjivar, Cecilia. 2011. *Enduring Violence: Ladina Women's Lives in Guatemala*. Berkeley, CA: University of California Press. http://www.ucpress.edu/ebook.php?isbn=9780520948419.

Pessar, Patricia. 2005. "Women, Gender, and International Migration Across and Beyond the Americas: Inequalities and Limited Empowerment." Expert Group Meeting on International Migration and Development in Latin America and the Caribbean, November.

Pomeroy, Elizabeth. 2011. "On Grief and Loss." *Social Work* 56 (2): 101–5. https://doi.org/10.1093/sw/56.2.101.

Reimann, Allison. 2009. "Hope for the Future? The Asylum Claims of Women Fleeing Sexual Violence in Guatemala." *University of Pennsylvania Law Review* 157 (4): 1199–1262.

Romeva I Rueda, Raül. 2007. "Draft Report on the Murders of Women (Feminicides) in Central America and Mexico and the Role of the European Union in Fighting this Phenomenon," Committee on Women's Rights and Gender Equality. http://www.europarl.europa.eu/sides/getDoc.do?type=COMPARL&mode=XML&language=EN&reference=PE388.414</Commission> Google Scholar.

Rosenblum, Marc, and Kate Brick. 2011. "U.S. Immigration Policy and Mexican/Central American Migration Flows: Then and Now." Migrationpolicy.org. 2011. https://www.migrationpolicy.org/research/RMSG-us-immigration-policy-mexican-central-american-migration-flows.

Salcido, Olivia, and Madelaine Adelman. 2004. "'He Has Me Tied with the Blessed and Damned Papers': Undocumented-Immigrant Battered Women in Phoenix, Arizona." *Human Organization* 63 (2): 162–72.

Salcioglu, Ebru, Sevim Urhan, Tugba Pirinccioglu, and Sule Aydin. 2017. "Anticipatory Fear and Helplessness Predict PTSD and Depression in Domestic Violence Survivors." *Psychological Trauma: Theory, Research, Practice and Policy* 9 (1): 117–25. https://doi.org/10.1037/tra0000200.

Steel, Zachary, Shakeh Momartin, Catherine Bateman, Atena Hafshejani, Derrick M. Silove, Naleya Everson, Konya Roy, et al. 2004. "Psychiatric Status of Asylum Seeker Families Held for a Protracted Period in a Remote Detention Centre in Australia." *Australian and New Zealand Journal of Public Health* 28 (6): 527–36.

Storm, Tania, and Marianne Engberg. 2013. "The Impact of Immigration Detention on the Mental Health of Torture Survivors Is Poorly Documented—a Systematic Review." *Danish Medical Journal* 60 (11): A4728.

Supin, Jeanne. 2016. "The Long Shadow: Bruce Perry on the Lingering Effects of Childhood Trauma." *The Sun*.

United Nations. 1993. Declaration on the Elimination of Violence against Women. New York: United Nations General Assembly.

———. 2004. Integration of the Human Rights of Women and a Gender Perspective: Violence against Women. *Report of the Special Rapporteur on violence against women, its causes and consequences*. Geneva, Switzerland.

Upegui-Hernández, Débora. 2012. "I. What Is Missing in the Transnational Migration Literature? A Latin American Feminist Psychological Perspective." *Feminism & Psychology* 22 (2): 228–39. https://doi.org/10.1177/0959353511415831.

Viola, Joelza M. A. Pires, and Rodrigo Grassi-Oliveira. 2014. "Mothers Who Were Sexually Abused during Childhood Are More Likely to Have a Child Victim of Sexual Violence." *Trends in Psychiatry and Psychotherapy* 36 (2): 119–22. https://doi.org/10.1590/2237-6089-2013-0054. Wagner, Heike. 2009. "Migration Und Gewalt Gegen Frauen. Über Unsichtbare Migrationsgründe Und Neuverhandlungen Im Migrationsprozess." *Anthropos* 104 (1): 41–61.

Wearick-Silva, Luis Eduardo, Saulo G. Tractenberg, Mateus L. Levandowski, Thiago W.

Chapter Ten

Access to Health Care, Institutional Violence, and Resistance of Female Transgender Sex Workers in Belo Horizonte, Brazil

Marco Aurélio Prado and Reynel Chaparro

Resistance studies have focused on the collective or institutional actions of groups facing several forms of oppression.[1] However, there are simultaneously different forms of individual resistances due to interactive and complex contexts of conflict. In this chapter, our main goal is to understand how the individual resistances of female transgender (trans) sex workers are interconnected with access to health care in different moments in Belo Horizonte, Brazil. As a result of qualitative data analysis of interviews on topics related to health-care access for trans sex workers, we recognize that segregation, prejudice, and ignorance of trans normativity by public institutions require for trans people in situ individual actions that guarantee (even if precariously in some cases) access to medical care in different interactions, oriented to reduce the negative experiences within the health-care system. Trans people demanding access to health-care systems show us the prevalence of exclusion and violence in public health-care institutions as well as the possibilities of individual actions to confront and modify this scenario. This chapter describes the trajectory of those strategies in different moments of health-care access.

ACCESS TO HEALTH CARE FOR TRANS SEX WORKERS IN BRAZIL

For trans people, the ideal health-care system connects their specific needs—which are oriented to counseling in hormone therapy, affirmative surgeries, and psychosocial care for them, their families, and their communities—with the usual ordinary, not compulsory, and specific health-care needs. This ideal involves sensitive health-care professionals that understand the impact of cisgendernormative (the supposition that everyone is cisgender) and heteronormative (the supposition that everyone is heterosexual) schemas in their practices, especially those with explicit and implicit sexual/gender binarism in their institutions. Guidelines for competent trans-affirmative care and inclusive attendance in health-care systems reflect the efforts of various health professionals and trans advocacy organizations to achieve a better understanding of the trans community and their needs in the health-care system (see Coleman et al. 2012; Hembree et al. 2018; Telfer, Tolit, Pace, & Pang 2018).

There are several indicators related to a trans-inclusive approach to health care, particularly the recognition of stigma and discrimination,[2] that includes cisgenderism; avoidance of trans preferred name or pronoun usage; inappropriate questions about trans corporeality; and assuming inherent mental instability, psychiatric issues,[3,4] and psychopathology[5,6] with mental health consequences for trans people in depression,[7] attempts and suicidal ideation,[8,9,10,11] and self-harm behavior.[12,13,14] Other indicators include suicide (Bauer, Pyne, Francino, & Hammond 2013; van Kesteren, Asscheman, Megens, & Gooren 1997) and high prevalence of HIV and other sexually transmitted diseases (Baral 2013).

Institutional violence that includes lack of explicit health care (Grant et al. 2011; Socias et al. 2014) makes trans people avoid health-care services for fear of discrimination (Bauer et al. 2009), but also includes postponing appointment attendance due to anti-trans bias (Grant et al. 2011). Recognizing these processes of discrimination and exclusion in the Brazilian health-care system, the Brazilian Ministry of Health, with its longstanding collaborative work with LGBT communities and advocates in health-care-specific needs, started the "Transexualization Process" (TP) (Brasil 2008a; Brasil 2008b) in the Unified Health System (UHS), a public policy created to assist trans people in their corporal modifications through the public health-care system.

Explicitly recognizing gender identity and sexual orientation, Brazilian health-care normativity includes a non-discriminatory stance with alerts about restriction or denial of health services, with specific indications about the use of "social name—name of" preference with trans clients, avoiding any forms of disrespect and prejudice for them (Brasil 2009). Other normative updates include, even in a pathological perspective, medical interventions for trans males (Conselho Federal de Medicina 2010), the inclusion of other identities such as transvestites and transsexuals in the TP, access to hormone therapy, clinical attendance and psychotherapy with or without affirmative surgeries, and geographical extensions with administrative health-care regulations that include TP access in primary care (Brasil 2013).

Rigid roles and behaviors associated with the concepts of masculinity and femininity as well as the assumption of heterosexuality (Lionço 2009) are some of the foremost criticisms of the TP. Still centered mainly in a pathological perspective (gender dysphoria) with a focus on corporal modifications, the TP is viewed as a new way to "regulate the sexuality" (Cardoso & Ferro 2012). This way of understanding trans clinical attendance prevents reflexive re-conceptualizations of health care that include other demands of the trans population beyond psychiatrization of care.

Despite the militancy and advocacy of trans social movements that collaborated on the elaboration and effectiveness of public policies oriented to trans, transvestites, and transsexual peoples (Lionço 2009), we recognize that there are still situations of rights restrictions at the individual and collective level. This political situation demands from trans people different actions to illuminate the implementation efforts of social programs in the health-care system that concern them.

RESISTANCE ACTIONS AS A FORM OF INTERACTION WITHIN DYNAMIC OPPRESSIVE CONTEXTS

Although there have been different attempts to categorize the resistance phenomenon (Williams 2009; Hollander & Einwohner 2004; Courpasson & Vallas 2016), we agree that maintaining an open mind to the lived experiences of people in different situations of oppression leads them to take different actions (conscious or not) as a response to dealing with different contextual oppressive structures. From this perspective of affirmation and personal agency, we can understand the different moments, emphases, and experiences of oppressed people beyond the application of normativity and sophisticated structures of the implementation of power (for example, Foucault's perspective of power or Tilly's organizations that influence policies and power dynamics).

According to Juris and Sitrin (2016), the phenomenon of resistance is complex and therefore requires a broad perspective for understanding that includes its different manifestations, dynamics, and particularities. An open perspective on the phenomenon of the resistance of oppressed people allows us to separate the binary perspective of an oppressive system versus an oppressed person. It allows us to be sensitive to the unique characteristics of the people and their differing ways of dealing with complex adverse situations. For this study, this involves different dynamics that are intertwined at the time of access to health care for trans people and includes the progressive implementation of public health policies oriented toward their access and specific needs.

The intersection of medical knowledge with specific normativity updates oriented to trans people that includes trans advocacy groups, strategic political actions, and demands of trans people in the context of health care is an interactive process that generates tensions, with different possibilities for people that demand an explicit attendance in the health-care system. With this in mind, one question arises: how do people act in the face of the conflicts that emerge in the context of demanding health services with a changing normativity that determines the possibilities of health care for trans people? We propose as a main focus of this study to describe and understand the different actions of resistance of trans people at the moment of access to public health care in Brazil.

METHODS

With data from an extensive ongoing research study titled, "Gender Identities and Repertoires of Psychopolitics Actions of Transvestites and Female Transsexuals Against Transphobic Violence" validated by Brazil's National Council for Scientific and Technological Development, we selected fourteen interviews of trans sex workers (between the ages of twenty-two and thirty-nine years old) from the city and metropolitan area of Belo Horizonte, Minas Gerais, Brazil, collected between 2011 and 2015. With the conformation of a team of three independent judges with experience in sexual and gender diversities, we conducted a qualitative multiple-case analysis through first approximation to the interviews with an open coding inductive analysis (Strauss 1987) on two topics: access to health care and UHS attendance.

Three subsequent meetings with the team were held to discuss the revision of the individual categories, as well as to establish categories around the actions of resistance of trans people in the health-care system and to try to identify a temporal sequence of how these categories emerge in different moments of access to health care. Sequential analytical networks were developed (Miles, Huberman, & Saldaña 2014) during the analysis of the categories. These networks were continually adjusted during the deliberative process and the analysis of new categories. This analytical strategy allows us to describe the trajectory and actions of resistance of trans people before, during, and after access to health.

FINDINGS AND DISCUSSION

Common elements are identified in the warning signs regarding self-perception of health status, which include changes in the body and symptoms that eventually trigger a search for help. At this moment, a reflection on the administrative aspects related to procedures, identity, and documentation to initiate the access to health care is activated, in some cases resulting in the participants remembering constraints and difficult situations in the UHS:

> "Look, even when I'm still being embarrassed by them, I'm going to the health clinic. And I took the identity card. That green identification card that in the UHS did not work at all. It's a joke. Because they ask for your identity card. Because I think that identity card has to be valid as a person's identity, right? But no, when I did not have Luciana's[15] identity I would take the other one, but I had to carry my identity card with my baptismal name."

> "[And you never looked for a health clinic here?] No! I do not seek a health clinic here because I do not even know where it is. But it's not because of being embarrassed. . . . I wanted to change my social name a while ago. Oh, what a peace! Several friends have already done this and I keep messing up! Here in Belo Horizonte is easy, easy. . ."

From this reflexive point, two sequences of access to health are identified. The first one is related with the identity card. Both reports indicate that despite the normativity that recognizes the social name in the health-care system (Brasil 2009) there is still an embarrassment in the use of the name on the registry in the health services.

Aspects of practicality and income (a socioeconomic aspect) trigger a series of strategies linked to activating a supportive network, which includes family members, friends, people from the circle of coexistence, and employees from the health-care network, which can advise in the search for care, follow up on consultations, as well as make it possible to link with the health system in different ways.

> "I had a very inflamed sore throat with blood coming out. I could not speak, and then my father said: "I am with my daughter, who is not my daughter, is my son, he has that name of his identity, but he likes to call himself Clarice because she's transsexual." And I kept thinking "How does he know I'm a transsexual?" I had not had this conversation with him, only with my mother. He talked a lot that I was going to become a woman, a transvestite, these things, but I think he saw that so much in the media. My father said: "We want a general practitioner to see us. Make the record and put it, Clarice, please." I had no problem because my father was there with me the first time and after that, I did it alone, I did it by myself."

After checking out symptoms, and remembering the context lived in the health-care system, often the easiest information available to reduce the symptoms is chosen, such as searching the internet (depending on access to technology); asking someone trustworthy in non-institutionalized environments that have a link with health, such as the pharmacy; self-medication; and searching for a private medical service (outside the UHS) that guarantees quick appointments and sensitivity to specific problems (for example sexually transmitted diseases). The higher cost for a private practice is associated with a legitimate demand for quality:

> "Ah my dear, in private (practice), if the *macho* knocks me out, I'll knock him out because I'm paying! (I pay for my bills) which come every month here to my house, and they have an obligation to treat me well."

A second sequence is directed towards the search for care in UHS, in which knowledge of the normative is involved as well as income and socioeconomics. We identified a request for attendance that generates a positive institutional response and a positive perception of trans people. On the other hand, institutional violence such as non-recognition of specific health-care normativity of trans identity is seen:

> "I was there (in the UHS) taking a girl from my house and she was called by the male name. Even me also, they called me by the male name. It was ridiculous, it was terrible, it was embarrassing, it was shameful, it was humiliating, I will not go back there again!"

Prejudice associated with HIV/AIDS:

> ". . . although it is not a specific area for the flu, because a transvestite also has the flu, we can have anything! We often say that the (trans) person has pain in the nail and they (healthcare providers) send us to take an AIDS test. So, they stereotype transvestites and AIDS."

Bureaucracy and the intrusive curiosity of health-care providers:

> "And the clinic, (trans) people avoid going too much because they have this form of prejudice. You go to a clinic and everybody wants to look at you, everyone wants to see you. You turn into the object of laughter for the nurses. Then you think you're a corpse that everyone can come and stick his or her hands on you, looking at you, calling the medical board, the academic nurses, everybody to scramble in to us. Then, I did what they do not want me to do. I took self-medication."

These situations trigger several responses, including indifference:

> "[You never feel embarrassed?] No, I'm not worried about that. I do not care too much."

Naturalization of violence:

> "I hit my head on the wall once and I spent time hearing buzzing, I ran to the clinic for care and I stayed there for hours, I did not receive any attendance and then I left."

Re-signification of prejudice:

> "It's not my case, because I'm not going there anymore (to UHS), I already went there (to UHS) and it did not work. It was not because of prejudice, but because of service."

Direct confrontation:

> ". . . at the time in the lobby (main entrance of UHS), I went to identify myself, there the girl asked me, 'What's your name?' and I said, 'Bruna, I came to visit my mother who is in the hospital.' . . . 'Ah, can you show me your identity card?' Then, I went and got my document, which was with the male name. 'Oh, but you've got your wrong identity card.' . . . 'It's not that way, you write Bruna that is, I'm already going!' 'Ah, but I do not know what I do not know. . . .' I didn't even look at her again, and I just went inside."

Insistence of attendance:

> "I received attendance only because I fought, only because I insisted and fought a lot. I say the same thing to people, everything has to be a fight, a discussion, an imposition, and you have to demand. . . . Something that should be natural only happens if it is because of the fight. I have suffered prejudice and discrimination, yes."

And avoidance of UHS:

> "Because a lot of time we often do not look there (UHS) because we know that there we will not be well attended, you know it will be annoying, embarrassing."

Prior to accessing institutionalized health care, some action strategies are identified that can be understood as ways of resisting the assistance that comes from institutional contexts and their knowledge about trans health.

This initial reaction is mediated by self-perception of health status, income, and practicality, where trans people can access relevant information more easily through non-institutionalized scenarios (internet and pharmacy).

Avoidance of the institutionalized health system appears as a compilation of negative experiences that have been experienced by trans people and shared through the dynamics of socialization, as part of the supportive social network that activates (or not) different options in the initial search for specific health-care demands (institutionalized—public vs. private—or outside of this context) (see figure 10.1). Concerns about the knowledge of specific regulations in health care that involve the recognition of their trans identity (with or without the identity card) is something that mediates the selection (or not) of entering institutional health-care environments.

On the other hand, the greatest difficulties in access to health and therefore where there is a greater repertoire of action strategies to face these difficulties by trans people is in the UHS, the context where specific normativity of attendance to trans people has been developed. The actions deployed by trans people are presented as a response to the different forms of institutional violence that is activated from the very first moment of a request for attendance and persist along the initial stages of intervention (see figure 10.2).

Actions by trans people can be understood at different levels ranging from less confrontation (indifference and naturalization of violence) to a reflective process that tries to weigh the situation of violence in intermediate terms (re-signification of prejudice), to a greater confrontation that becomes more noticeable and directed towards the different actors of institutional violence (confrontation and insistence of attendance). Avoiding the use of UHS seems to be a differentiated response that can be understood as an act of resistance, a way of opposing the violence that is experienced in the UHS.

Acceptance, proper treatment, and positive perception of access and attendance in health care helps trans people returning to the health-care system with adherence and continuity in treatment. On the other hand, all the negative elements that we identified in the UHS create the avoidance of UHS. Both identified sequences of action are characterized by the perception of the severity of the symptoms and the level of controllability and responses that each action has in the perception of well-being.

The choice between private and public health-care systems is based on the interaction of different factors, such as income and supportive social networks, as well as the possibility of a quick response by the institutions to their health demands. According to some trans people, long waiting times at receptions and lineups are contexts of embarrassment, due to the different types of violence experienced in these spaces, such as whispers or comments about them, inquisitive looks, and insults from other people there. With the

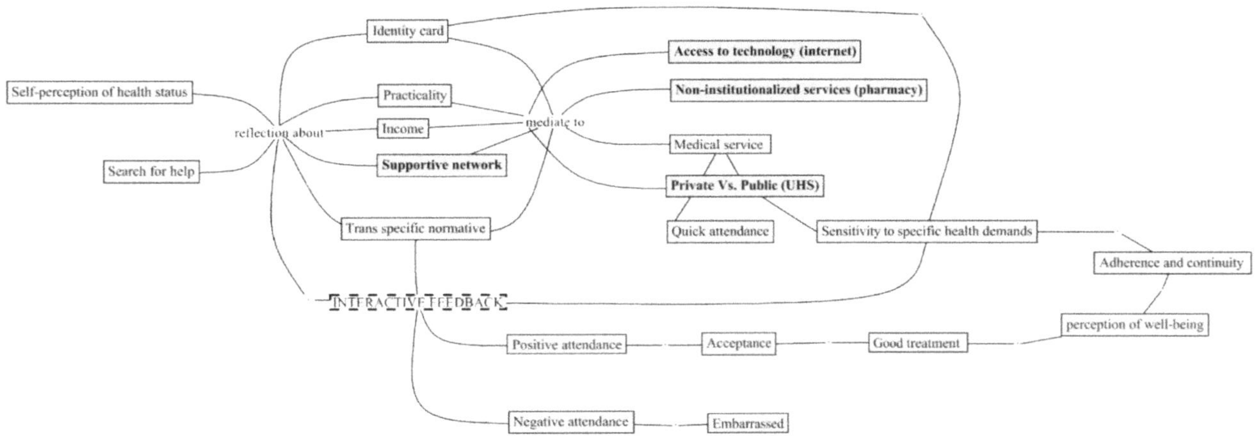

Figure 10.1. Diagrammatic representation of the dynamic process of access to health care.
Figure created by authors

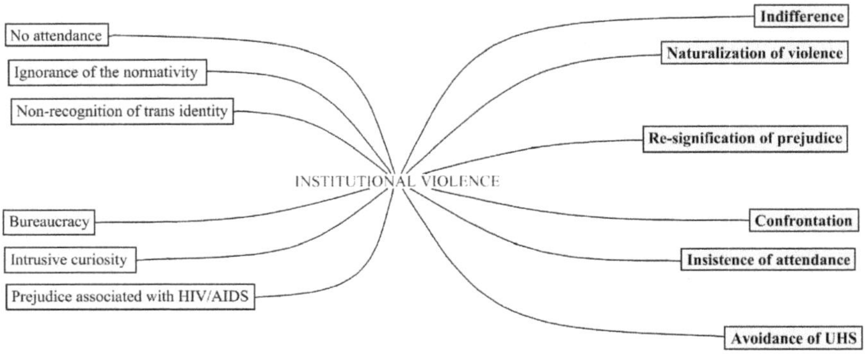

Figure 10.2. Institutional violence and resistance actions along the initial stages of access to health care.
Figure created by authors

perception of a welcoming, faster, and more effective service, the treatment is well-evaluated and increases a positive perception of the health-care experience, thus facilitating adherence (see figure 10.1). However, the use of the private health system demands greater financial expenses, often outside the range of possibility for trans people, who are largely in an extreme situation of social and economic vulnerability.

FINAL CONSIDERATIONS

As a fragile moment in the experiences of trans people, access to the health-care system is a necessary condition for adherence and permanence; it is the materialization of the right to be healthy in the context of respectful care and attendance. The analysis of actions related to access to the health-care system by trans people shows us the importance of primary care, especially in public versus private services. For trans people, primary care is an open door or certainly a big wall to climb, even with an updated normativity structure that tries to generate an inclusive strategy to facilitate their access to health care in the Brazilian public health-care system.

Bureaucracy and the difficulties related to identifying the clients in the heteronormative–cisgender schema show us the violence directed toward recognition of the social name of trans people, an initial obstacle that requires differential actions that influence the dynamics of the health-care system. In this context, many strategies on an individual and collective level can be considered as part of a repertoire of actions that create resistances in particular ways and share some practices in a conflictive context from memories and feelings of injustice from different political conflicts. Looking from this perspective is to understand how the public health-care services in Brazil can transform health-care practices to better assist transgender people.

NOTES

1. We are very grateful to the trans sex workers who participated in this project, who allowed us access to their experiences in the health-care system. We also thank Lohana Morelli and Bárbara Gonçalves from the Federal University of Minas Gerais for their participation as judges in the process of data analysis and their helpful comments in the first steps of this research.
2. Harper & Schneider 2003.
3. Lefkowitz & Mannell 2017.
4. Snelgrove, Jasudavisius, Rowe, Head, & Bauer 2012.
5. Nadal, Rivera, & Corpus 2010.
6. Nadal, Skolnik, & Wong 2012.
7. Rotondi, Bauer, Travers, & Travers 2011.
8. Clements-Nolle, Marx, & Katz 2006.
9. Cochran & Cauce 2006.
10. Nuttbrock et al. 2010.
11. Xavier et al. 2005.
12. Dickey, Reisner, & Juntunen 2015.
13. Goldblum et al., 2012.
14. Testa et al. 2012.
15. With the purpose of preserving anonymity all names have been changed.

WORKS CITED

American Psychological Association. (2015). "Guidelines for psychological practice with transgender and gender non-conforming people." *American Psychologist*, 70(9): 832–864. https://doi.com/10.1037/a0039906.

Baral, S. D., Poteat, T., Strömdahl, S., Wirtz, A. L., Guadamuz, T. T. & Beyrer, C. (2013). "Worldwide burden of HIV in transgender women: a systematic review and meta-analysis." *The Lancet Infectious Diseases*, 13(3): 214–222. https://doi.com/10.1016/S1473-3099(12)70315-8.

Bauer, G. R., Hammond, R., Travers, R., Kaay, M., Hohenadel, K. M. & Boyce, M. (2009). "'I don't think this is theoretical; this is our lives': How erasure impacts health care for transgender people." *Journal of the Association of Nurses in AIDS Care*, 20(5): 348–361. https://doi.com/10.1016/j.jana.2009.07.004.

Bauer, G. R., Pyne, J., Francino, M. C. & Hammond, R. (2013). "La suicidabilité parmi les personnes trans en Ontario: implications en travail social et en justice sociale." *Service Social*, 59: 35–62. https://doi.com/10.7202/1017478ar.

Brasil. (2008a). "Portaria GM nº 1707, de 18 de agosto de 2008. Institui, no âmbito do Sistema Único de Saúde (SUS), o Processo Transexualizador, a ser implantado nas unidades federadas, respeitadas as competências das três esferas de gestão." Ministério da Saúde.

Brasil. (2008b). "Portaria nº 457, de 19 de agosto de 2008." Ministério da Saúde. Secretaria de Atenção à Saúde.

Brasil. (2009). "Portaria MS nº 1.820, de 13 de agosto de 2009. Dispõe sobre os direitos e deveres dos usuários da saúde." Ministério da Saúde.

Brasil. (2013). "Portaria nº 2.803, de 19 de novembro de 2013. Redefine e amplia o Processo Transexualizador no Sistema Único de Saúde (SUS)." Ministério da Saúde.

Cardoso, M. R. & Ferro, L. F. (2012). "Saúde e população LGBT: demandas e especificidades em questão." *Psicologia: Ciência e Profissão*, 32(3): 552–563. https://doi.com/10.1590/S1414-98932012000300003.

Clements-Nolle, K., Marx, R. & Katz, M. (2006). "Attempted suicide among transgender persons: The influence of gender-based discrimination and victimization." *Journal of Homosexuality*, 51: 53–69. https://doi.com/10.1300/J082v51n03_04.

Cochran, B. N. & Cauce, A. M. (2006). "Characteristics of lesbian, gay, bisexual, and transgender individuals entering substance abuse treatment." *Journal of Substance Abuse Treatment*, 30: 135–146. https://doi.com/10.1016/j.jsat.2005.11.009.

Coleman, E., Bockting, W., Botzer, M., Cohen-Kettenis, P., DeCuypere, G. Feldman, J., Fraser, L., et al. (2012). "Standards of care for the health of transsexual, transgender, and gender-nonconforming people," version 7. *International Journal of Transgenderism*, 13(4): 165–232. https://doi.com/10.1080/15532739.2011.700873.

Conselho Federal de Medicina. (2010). "Resolução n. 1.955, de 3 de setembro de 2010. Dispõe sobre a cirurgia de transgenitalismo e revoga a Resolução CFM n. 1.652, de 2 de dezembro de 2002."

Courpasson, D. & Vallas, S. (2016). "Resistance studies. A critical introduction." In D. Courpasson, & S. Vallas (Eds.). *The SAGE Handbook of Resistance* (1–28). London, GB: SAGE. https://doi.com/10.4135/9781473957947.n1.

Dickey, l. m., Reisner, S. L. & Juntunen, C. L. (2015). "Non-suicidal self-injury in a large online sample of transgender adults." *Professional Psychology: Research and Practice*, 46: 3–11. https://doi.com/10.1037/a0038803.

Goldblum, P., Testa, R. J., Pflum, S., Hendricks, M. L., Bradford, J. & Bongar, B. (2012). "In-school gender-based victimization and suicide attempts in transgender individuals." *Professional Psychology: Research and Practice*, 43: 468–475. https://doi.com/10.1037/a0029605.

Grant, J. M., Mottet, L. A., Tanis, J., Harrison, J., Herman, J. L. & Keisling, M. (2011). "Injustice at every turn: A report of the National Transgender Discrimination Survey." Washington: *National Center for Transgender Equality and National Gay and Lesbian Task Force*. Available in: http://www.thetaskforce.org/static_html/downloads/reports/reports/ntds_full.pdf.

Harper, G. & Schneider, M. (2003). "Oppression and discrimination among lesbian, gay, bisexual and transgender people and communities: A challenge for community psychology." *American Journal of Community Psychology*, 31(3–4): 243–252. https://doi.com/10.1023/A:1023906620085.

Hembree, W. C., Cohen-Kettenis, P. T., Gooren, L., Hannema, S. E., Meyer, W. J., Murad, M. H., Rosenthal S. M., et al. (2017). "Endocrine treatment of gender-dysphoric/gender-incongruent persons: An endocrine society clinical practice guideline." *Journal of Clinical Endocrinology & Metabolism*, 102: 3869–3903. doi:10.1210/jc.2017-01658.

Hollander, J. A. & Einwohner, R. L. (2004). "Conceptualizing resistance." *Sociological Forum*, 19(4): 533–554. https://doi.com/10.1007/s11206-004-0694-5.

Juris, J. & Sitrin, M. (2016). "Globalization, Resistance, and Social Transformation." In D. Courpasson, & S. Vallas (Eds.). *The SAGE Handbook of Resistance* (31–50). London, GB: SAGE. https://doi.com/10.4135/9781473957947.n2.

Lefkowitz, A. & Mannell, J. (2017). "Sexual health service providers' perceptions of transgender youth in England." *Health and Social Care in the Community*, 25(3): 1237–1246. https://doi.com/10.1111/hsc.12426.

Lionço, T. (2009). "Atenção integral à saúde e diversidade sexual no Processo Transexualizador do SUS: Avanços, impasses, desafios." *Physis Revista de Saúde Coletiva*, 19(1): 43–63. https://doi.com/10.1590/S0103-73312009000100004.

Miles, M.B., Huberman, A.M. & Saldaña, J. (2014). *Qualitative data analysis: A methods sourcebook*. Sage, London.

Nadal, K. L., Rivera, D. P. & Corpus, M. J. H. (2010). "Sexual orientation and transgender microaggressions in everyday life: Experiences of lesbians, gays, bisexuals, and transgender individuals." In D. W. Sue (Ed.), *Microaggressions and marginality: Manifestation, dynamics, and impact* (217–240). New York, NY: Wiley.

Nadal, K. L., Skolnik, A. & Wong, Y. (2012). "Interpersonal and systemic microaggressions toward transgender people: Implications for counseling." *Journal of LGBT Issues in Counseling*, 6(1): 55–82. https://doi.com/10.1080/15538605.2012.648583.

Nuttbrock, L., Hwahng, S., Bockting, W., Rosenblum, A., Mason, M., Macri, M. & Becker, J. (2010). "Psychiatric impact of gender-related abuse across the life course of male-to-female transgender persons." *Journal of Sex Research*, 47: 12–23. https://doi.com/10.1080/00224490903062258.

Rotondi, N. K., Bauer, G. R., Travers, R. & Travers, A. (2011). "Depression in male-to-female transgender Ontarians: results from the Trans PULSE Project." *Canadian Journal of Community Mental Health*. 30(2): 113–133. https://doi.com/10.7870/cjcmh-2011-0020.

Snelgrove, J. D., Jasudavisius, A. M., Rowe, B. W., Head, E. M. & Bauer, G. R. (2012). "'Completely out-at-sea'" with 'two-gender medicine': A qualitative analysis of physician-side barriers to providing health care for transgender patients." *BMC Health Services Research*, 12: 110. https://doi.com/10.1186/1472-6963-12-110.

Socias, M. E., Marshall, B. D. L., Aristegui, I., Romero, M., Cahn, P., Kerr, T. & Sued, O. (2014). "Factors associated with healthcare avoidance among transgender women in Argentina." *International Journal for Equity in Health*, 13(1): 81. https://doi.com/10.1186/s12939-014-0081-7.

Strauss, A. L. (1987). *Qualitative analysis for social scientists*. New York, NY, US: Cambridge University Press. https://doi.com/10.1017/CBO9780511557842.

Telfer, M.M., Tollit, M.A., Pace, C.C., & Pang, K.C. (2018). "Australian standards of care and treatment guidelines for trans and gender diverse children and adolescents" Version 1.1. The Royal Children's Hospital. Melbourne. Available at: https://www.rch.org.au/uploadedFiles/Main/Content/adolescent-medicine/australian-standards-of-care-and-treatment-guidelines-for-trans-and-gender-diverse-children-and-adolescents.pdf.

Testa, R. J., Sciacca, L. M., Wang, F., Hendricks, M. L., Goldblum, P., Bradford, J. & Bongar, B. (2012). "Effects of violence on transgender people." *Professional Psychology: Research and Practice*, 43: 452–459. https://doi.com/10.1037/a0029604.

van Kesteren, P. J. M., Asscheman, H., Megens, J. O. J. & Gooren, L. J. G. (1997). "Mortality and morbidity in transsexual subjects treated with cross-sex hormones." *Clinical Endocrinology*, 47: 337–342. https://doi.com/10.1046/j.1365-2265.1997.2601068.x.

Williams, J. P. (2009). "The multidimensionality of resistance in youth-subcultural studies." *The Resistance Studies Magazine*, 1: 20–33.

Xavier, J., Bobbin, M., Singer, B. & Budd, E. (2005). "A needs assessment of transgendered people of color living in Washington, DC." *International Journal of Transgenderism*, 8: 31–47. https://doi.com/10.1300/ J485v08n02_04.

Index

About the Contributors

Shir Lerman Ginzburg, PhD, MPH, is a project director in the Department of Pediatrics and the Preventive Intervention Research Center for Child Health (PIRC) at the Albert Einstein College of Medicine. Her research interests currently focus on mental health outcomes among K-12 students in public school students in the Bronx. She is trained as a medical anthropologist and public health professional, and has conducted research in syndemics, chronic illness, mental health, obesity, diabetes, mindfulness, the Zika virus, Puerto Rico, and the United States. She received her PhD in medical anthropology from the University of Connecticut, where she identified a new syndemic in Puerto Rico: the OVIDD Syndemic (Obesity, structural Violence, political Instability, Diabetes, and Depression). She completed her NIH-funded post-doctoral fellowship in implementation science at the University of Massachusetts Medical School, where she studied the correlation between mindfulness and mental health outcomes among underserved communities in the greater Boston area. She has coedited two books, *Foundations of BioSocial Health: Stigma and Illness Interactions* and *Stigma Syndemics: New Directions in BioSocial Health*, and has also published research articles in journals such as *Medical Anthropology*, *Medical Anthropology Theory*, and *PLOS One*.

Ronnie Anthony Shepard, PhD, regularly teaches courses in anthropology, gender and sexuality studies, and Latin American studies at universities throughout New England. He is a former editor of *Ariel*, the annual newsletter of El Instituto: The Center for Latin American and Caribbean Studies at the University of Connecticut. Prior to his work in higher education and as a cultural anthropologist, he spent five years running and designing collaborative programming as one of the co-founders of the Among Men/For Men drop-in center and peer support group at Tapestry Health of Western Massachusetts.

Working with marginalized populations at Tapestry took him in several directions including community outreach work among MSM and substance abusing populations and HIV/AIDS case management. He also helped organize local events including the Black HIV/AIDS Awareness Dinner and acted as master of ceremonies for the Western Massachusetts edition of the Bayard Rustin Community Breakfast. Today, his research interests continue to lie with marginalized gender and sexual populations in Latin America, as well as domestic minority/underrepresented populations in higher education settings. After studying abroad as an undergraduate and with over a decade of ethnographic research in the streets of Quito, he considers Ecuador his home away from home.

Shan-Estelle Brown is a medical anthropologist and assistant professor of anthropology at Rollins College where she co-coordinates the Global Health Program. Previously, she was a postdoctoral researcher in the AIDS Program at Yale School of Medicine. Her research articulates patient experiences in clinical settings for chronic diseases like HIV, substance use, and sickle cell disease. She holds a doctorate in anthropology from the University of Connecticut, a master's of arts in English from Old Dominion University, and a Bachelor of Arts in Humanities from Yale University. She is the author of *Writing in Anthropology: A Brief Guide* published by Oxford University Press.

Reynel Chaparro, MSc, PhD, is a social psychologist from the National University of Colombia (Colciencias Scholarship 647–2014). He created the student group Psychological Intervention and Sexual Diversity at the National University of Colombia, in which community intervention projects were developed on topics related to sexual orientations, gender identities, and the link between religion/spirituality and sexual/gender diversity. His work has been focused on the understanding of sexual and gender diversities, as well as LGBTQI+ identities and their dynamics in different contexts of health intervention in both Colombia and Brazil. Since 2016, he has been the Colombian College of Psychologists' (*Colegio Colombiano de Psicologós* COLPSIC) representative for the International Psychology Network for Lesbian, Gay, Bisexual, Transgender and Intersex Issues (IPsyNet) of the American Psychological Association (APA).

Laurie Cook Heffron, PhD, LMSW, is an assistant professor in the School of Behavioral and Social Sciences at St. Edward's University in Austin, Texas, where she teaches undergraduate students and directs the Social Work Field Education Program. She joined the faculty of St. Edward's University after having served as Post-Doctoral Fellow in Immigration and Violence Against Women at the University of Texas at Austin and as former Associate Director for Research at UT-Austin's Institute on Domestic Violence and Sexual

Assault. Cook Heffron's research and expertise focus on domestic and sexual violence, human trafficking, and the experiences of, and relationships between, violence against women and migration. She also draws from direct social work practice experience with a variety of communities, including refugees, asylum-seekers, trafficked persons, and other immigrants. Blending her research and practice experience, she regularly provides assessments and serves as an expert witness in immigration cases of women and children seeking T visas, U visas, and asylum based on domestic violence. She studied linguistics and Spanish at Georgetown University and earned a master's degree in social work and a doctorate in social work from The University of Texas at Austin.

Evgenia Fotiou is a cultural anthropologist and an assistant professor of anthropology at Kent State University. She has a PhD in cultural anthropology and Latin American studies from the University of Wisconsin–Madison, where she completed doctoral research on Amazonian shamanism in Peru and its transformation through globalization and the formation of transnational tourist networks. She is interested in health and healing in cross-cultural perspective and is currently writing a book on Amazonian sorcery while researching the revitalization of pre-Christian religion in modern Greece. Fotiou is an expert in the anthropology of religion, shamanism, medical anthropology, Amazonian cultures, and gender, and teaches courses on these subjects. Her current work urges scholars of all disciplines to reexamine assumptions about indigenous knowledge systems and to engage meaningfully with non-Western epistemologies.

Adriana M. Garriga-López, PhD, is a cultural anthropologist and artist whose work focuses on epidemics and disasters as events that make visible the workings of colonial power, climate change, race, gender, and sexuality in the Caribbean. Garriga-López is associate professor of anthropology and chair of the Anthropology and Sociology Department at Kalamazoo College in Michigan. She is also associate faculty of the Brooklyn Institute for Social Research and serves on the board of directors of OutFront Kalamazoo, an organization serving the LGBTQ community of southwest Michigan.

Dora Gonzalez is a graduate student at the University of Texas at Austin pursuing a dual degree in master's of science in social work (MSSW) and master's of arts in Latin American studies. Her research interests include migration traumas and resiliency/coping mechanisms of asylum-seeking families from three Central American countries: Honduras, El Salvador, and Guatemala. Gonzalez is also a community organizer in Austin for immigrant and labor rights, and she currently serves on the board of directors of two area not-for-profits: Austin Tan Cerca de la Frontera, a coalition seeking to address conditions of social and economic injustice along the Texas/Mexico border and find community-driven alternatives through transnational solidarity and fair trade, and Justice for Our Neighbors–Austin Region, an immigration law office providing free, high-quality legal services.

Anayeli Marcos is a dual degree candidate at the University of Texas at Austin pursuing master's degrees in social work (MSSW) and Latin American studies (MA). She is currently an Integrated Behavioral Health (IBH) scholar and a research assistant at the Texas Institute for Child and Family Well-being. As a DACA recipient and activist, her research interests are focused on the immigrant community around topics of trauma and migration, social movements, gender-based violence, detention, forced migration, and parenting. Marcos's current research is seeking to explore the impact of trauma-informed care practices of lawyers and legal immigrant advocates working with unaccompanied minors. Upon the completion of her degrees, Marcos hopes to remain in Texas and continue creating, providing, and researching ways in which health providers can be better equipped to address the growing issues of immigrant families in the United States.

Olivia Marcus, MPH, is a PhD candidate in medical anthropology at the University of Connecticut. Her doctoral work considers the implications of therapeutic pluralism in the Peruvian Amazon for mental well-being among people who work with curanderos. Prior to her fieldwork in the Amazon, she worked as a public health professional at the New York Psychiatric Institute as project manager for a behavioral intervention to reduce risk of HIV transmission among juvenile justice youth. She has conducted research on health behaviors related to people living with HIV/AIDS in the United States and east Africa, ethnomedical beliefs concerning Ebola transmission in Cameroon, and the role of internet memes during an infectious disease epidemic.

Lauren M. Pérez-Bonilla is a PhD candidate in the Department of Geography at the University of Connecticut. An interdisciplinary scholar and researcher, she obtained her MA in international studies from the same institution in Spring 2018 and a BA in social sciences with a minor in International Relations from the University of Puerto Rico, Rio Piedras (UPR-RP). Her research interests include Dominican masculinities, Caribbean sex work(ers), neoliberal subjects in the Caribbean, geopolitics, and the (re)construction of space based on social memory. In addition to her role as a scholar, she is also a skilled photographer. In 2017, the Human Rights Institute (HRI) at UConn granted her the Robin Romano Award for Investigative Journalism to document the places where sex work takes place and the people who engage in it in the Dominican Republic. Her work has been featured in electronic magazines including *[in]Genios* and *Living Language*.

Marco Aurélio Prado is a psychologist and PhD in social psychology from Pontifical Catholic University of São Paulo (PUCSP). He is currently a professor at the Federal University of Minas Gerais (UFMG/Brazil) and is the coordinator of the LGBT Human Rights and Citizenship Research Group (NUH/UFMG). Prado is a professor at the Graduate Program in Social Psychology working with LGBTI issues and public policy, human rights and LGBT political actions, and transgender and public health in Brazil. In 1995, he was awarded a Fulbright Grant at the University of Massachusetts/Amherst. He is a member of the International Psychology Network for Lesbian, Gay, Bisexual, Transgender and Intersex Issues (Ipsynet) of the American Psychological Association (APA). Prado is the co-author of several books on topics including gender, homosexuality, transgender experience, social psychology perspectives, and political thoughts in political psychology.

Carlos E. Rodríguez-Díaz, PhD, MPH, MCHES, is associate professor in the Milken Institute School of Public Health at the George Washington University. He is a community health scientist with over fifteen years of experience conducting participatory research in Puerto Rico, the United States and the Caribbean Region. His work has focused on the areas of HIV care and prevention, sexual health promotion, and health equity through actions on the social determinants of health. Rodríguez-Díaz completed post-doctoral training in HIV and global health research, a PhD in public health with a major in community health, and an MPH in health education. He has also completed post-graduate training in health policy, human rights, and health diplomacy. He has contributed to projects funded by the Centers for Disease Control and Prevention, the National Institutes of Health, and the Health Resources and Services Administration, as well as private and not-for-profit organizations. He has published in major scientific journals including the *American Journal of Public Health*, *Journal of Sexual Medicine*, *Archives of Sexual Behavior*, and *Journal of Immigration and Minority Health*, among others.

Leyla Savloff is a doctoral candidate in the Department of Anthropology at the University of Washington. Her dissertation, "*Entre Mujeres:* The Social and Political Spheres of Women Against Prison," examines how a collective of formerly incarcerated women enact freedom through art practices and activism in contemporary Argentina. This research has been funded by the American Association of University Women's American Dissertation Fellowship, the Dr. Clyde Snow Fund for Latin American Studies, and the Latinx Scholars Graduate School Fellowship. Broadly, her research investigates women's collectives in Latin America that contest surveillance techniques and promote community-based approaches against institutional violence. She currently volunteers at University Beyond Bars and is a member of the Alliance for Higher Education in Prison.

Antwann Michael Simpkins is a PhD candidate in the Department of Sociology at the University of California, Los Angeles. His primary research interests are race, gender, law and society, and Black feminist thought. He is a Phi Beta Kappa graduate of Morehouse College and serves as a lecturer with both the Los Angeles Community College District and UCLA. Beyond his academic work, Simpkins is committed to the success of his students and enjoys mentoring them toward the goals they have set for themselves.

Tia Tyndal, BA, is the research coordinator of the Duke University Interdisciplinary Behavioral Research Center. She received her BA in psychology and women and gender studies from Florida International University. Her research interests focus mainly on suicide prevention and the treatment of self-injurious behaviors in adolescents. Currently, she is interested in the roles that social media and emerging technology play in influencing suicidal thoughts and self-injurious behaviors. She is also a Ronald E. McNair Scholar and participant in the Leadership Alliance who completed her research titled, "Measuring the Suicidal Mind: Can Behavioral Tests Predict Suicidal Thoughts and Behaviors" at Harvard University. She regularly holds conversations on social justice issues at her Dinner and Discussion gatherings in the Raleigh-Durham area.

Ana Vidina Hernández, MA, MSSW, is the program and research coordinator for Girasol at the Texas Institute for Child and Family Wellbeing in the School of Social Work at the University of Texas at Austin. Girasol engages with research and programming to support the immigrant community and immigrants in detention in the state of Texas. Hernández's research interests include immigration, the impacts of detention, trauma, domestic violence, sexual assault, and experiences of undocumented youth and young adults. She is also a trained social worker and a lead therapist at the YWCA Greater Austin, where she provides bilingual counseling services to individuals and families and facilitates a support group for immigrant women in detention. Her master's thesis at the UT Austin Lozano Long Institute of Latin American studies is titled "Becoming Undocumented and Unafraid: Impacts of 'Illegality' on Identity Formation and University Student Activism."

www.ingramcontent.com/pod-product-compliance
Ingram Content Group UK Ltd.
Pitfield, Milton Keynes, MK11 3LW, UK
UKHW020212290926
15470UKWH00001B/139

9 781498 572842